HIV & AIDS

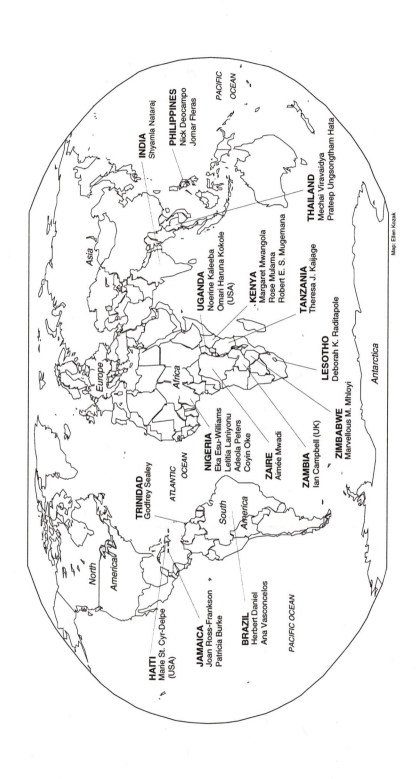

PACIFIC
OCEAN

INDIA
Shyamla Nataraj

PHILIPPINES
Nick Deocampo
Jomar Fleras

THAILAND
Mechai Viravaidya
Prateep Ungsongtham Hata

Asia

UGANDA
Noerine Kaleeba
Omari Haruna Kokole
(USA)

KENYA
Margaret Mwangola
Rose Mulama
Robert E. S. Mugemana

TANZANIA
Theresa J. Kajiage

Europe

Africa

LESOTHO
Deborah K. Raditapole

Antarctica

NIGERIA
Eka Esu-Williams
Letitia Laniyonu
Adeola Peters
Coyin Oke

ZAIRE
Aimée Mwadi

ZIMBABWE
Marvellous M. Mhloyi

ZAMBIA
Ian Campbell (UK)

TRINIDAD
Godfrey Sealey

ATLANTIC
OCEAN

South

America

North
America

HAITI
Marie St. Cyr-Delpe
(USA)

JAMAICA
Joan Ross-Frankson
Patricia Burke

BRAZIL
Herbert Daniel
Ana Vasconcelos

PACIFIC OCEAN

Map: Ellen Kozak

HIV & AIDS

The Global Inter-Connection

editor
Elizabeth Reid

Published in cooperation with the
United Nations Development Programme

Kumarian Press

Kumarian Press Books for a World that Works

HIV & AIDS: The Global Inter-Connection. Published 1995 in the United States of America by Kumarian Press, Inc., 14 Oakwood Avenue, West Hartford, Connecticut 06119-2127 USA.

Production supervised by Jenna Dixon
Text design by Jenna Dixon   *Copyedited by Linda Lotz*
Typeset by UltraGraphics   *Proofread by Jolene Robinson*
Index by Barbara DeGennaro

Printed in the United States of America on recycled acid-free paper by Edwards Brothers, Inc. Text printed with soy-based ink.

Library of Congress Cataloging-in-Publication Data
HIV & AIDS : the global inter-connection / editor, Elizabeth Reid ;
    United Nations Development Programme.
          p.   cm.   -- (Kumarian Press books for a world that works)
    Includes index.
    ISBN 1-56549-041-X (alk. paper)
    1. AIDS (Disease)—Social aspects. I. Reid, Elizabeth, 1942-
II. United Nations Development Programme. III. Title: HIV and
AIDS. IV. Series.
    RA644.A25H577   1995
    362.1'969792--dc20   94-43316

06 05 04 03 02 01 00 99 98 97   12 11 10 9 8 7 6 5 4 3

Contents

Foreword

During the last fifteen years, the human immunodeficiency virus (HIV) epidemic has entered our consciousness as an incomprehensible calamity, already laying claim to millions of human lives, inflicting grief and pain, causing uncertainty and fear, and threatening economic devastation. It poses serious problems everywhere for sustainable human development, but it is especially devastating for the countries of the developing world.

Eighty per cent of the world's population lives in the countries of the developing world. That is where an estimated 13 to 18 million people, mostly children, die from hunger, malnutrition, and poverty-related causes each year. In Africa, one in twenty-one women dies in pregnancy or childbirth; in Asia, one in fifty-four; in Latin America, one in seventy-three. For each of these women, another fifteen, 98 per cent of them in the developing world, become ill or disabled each year as a result of complications in childbearing.

One billion people live in households too poor to obtain the food necessary for sustaining normal work. Half a billion live in households too poor to obtain the food needed for minimal activity. One-third of all households in the developing world are headed by women and, by 1990, at least a quarter of the women heading households were elderly.

These are the countries where 80 per cent of new HIV infections are occurring, and it is estimated that by the year 2000, 90 per cent of all new infections will occur there. The havoc that could be wrought by the HIV epidemic, combined with these already existing conditions, is beyond the comprehension of most of us.

Despite the complexity of the causes and consequences of the HIV epidemic, people have been finding ways to respond. Individuals, families, villages, and communities are organizing and working together to support those affected, to assist the survivors, to help one another change behaviour in order to remain uninfected.

The United Nations Development Programme is committed to supporting these processes of change, which originate in the dreams and aspirations of affected people themselves. This book of personal reflections allows the voices of some of these individuals to be heard.

James Gustave Speth
Administrator
United Nations Development Programme

Preface

The origins of this book lay in a desire to stimulate people to think of the ways in which the human immunodeficiency virus (HIV) epidemic might affect their lives, their work and their communities in the years to come—a span of time similar to that which separates one generation from another. In what ways would their children be affected? How would it feel to live in their communities? Would the nature of their work be affected, its political setting, its economic base?

As we worked with the contributors, we discovered a striking fact about the epidemic. As one comes to live within this epidemic, one realizes that the future will not resemble the pre-HIV past. The virus is here in our midst. Change is now an imperative for survival. However, at this stage in our consciousness, there seems to be in each of us a deep reluctance, or an incapacity, to see the future.

And so what was to have been a book of reflections on its impact is now a book of reflections on the epidemic itself. It is also a book of reflections *of* the epidemic. The epidemic is a reflective surface. It throws into stark relief the fault lines of a society: the way power is exercised, gender constructed, socioeconomic stratification exploited; the moral ambiguities, the interpersonal slippages. But it also highlights the strengths: empathy, courage, compassion, commitment, intelligence, solidarity, faith. It makes us think, challenging us less with our mortality than with our living interdependence.

The voices you will hear in these pages come from a variety of backgrounds, experiences and concerns. They reflect where the virus has penetrated and what it has unearthed. Each has its point of view and its focus of concern. This gives the book texture and diversity. The thread that weaves through them is a sense of urgency and of passionate concern, even outrage against self and others that so little has yet been achieved, and so much remains to be done.

The voices are loosely organized in the book from the outward turning—the analyses of the settings of the epidemic and their impact on where and how quickly the virus is spreading—through the inward turning—the impact on self and loved ones—to the voices that are pointing out the paths we must travel, now and in the future.

These same voices also underscore the importance of language in describing and discussing the HIV epidemic. They have informed UNDP language policy and tell their own stories of how language can fuel intolerance and misunderstanding or, alternatively, foster compassion and acceptance.

In undertaking to bring this book about, UNDP wanted the voices of the developing world to be more widely heard, to be a part of the global activism. This book would not have been possible without the unstinting support—in time, encouragement and advocacy—of Timothy Rothermel, director of the Science, Technology and Private Sector Division within which the HIV and Development Programme is nested at UNDP.

In its inception, the book was guided by an advisory board consisting of Timothy Rothermel; Ingar Bruggermann, director of the World Health Organization's New

York liaison office; and Lloyd Garrison, Jehan Raheem, Frank Hartvelt and Mina Mauerstein-Bail of UNDP, who provided guidance on approach, suggested contributors and interviewers, and helped with the technicalities and formalities of the publishing world.

The initial management of the project was provided by the Ms. Foundation for Education and Communication, Inc. Its editorial team was directed by Marcia Gillespie as senior editor, who commissioned the writings on behalf of UNDP. The final editing was done by Kakuna Kerina, who brought her knowledge of her own newly independent country, Namibia, and of Africa in general to her work and enriched it and us. Under their guidance, the text has emerged as a blend of the public and the private, the subjective and the objective—a complexity that reflects that of the epidemic itself.

Special thanks are due to Mina Mauerstein-Bail, Michael Bailey, Kasia Malinowska, Darlene Chavis, Gail Learner and the other members of the HIV and Development Programme, past and present, who kept the project going despite their own demanding responsibilities. Berl Francis, Edison Maciel, George Orick and Wasant Techawongtham interviewed some of the contributors. Professor Norman Miller served as a consultant to the project in its final stages. Finally, Krishna Sondhi and Trish Reynolds of Kumarian Press are also to be thanked for their efforts in shepherding this book through the production process.

We would like to thank everyone who contributed their thoughts, whether or not their reflections were included in this volume. Each contributor gave new insights into this complex phenomenon that now faces the world. Our work is the richer. Their insights appear in our writings; their ideas guide us.

Finally, we would like to thank Bill, Brett, Bill, Noerine, Troy and his dad Vince, Stephen, Cindi, Mianda, Auxilla, David, Michael, Robert, Herbert and many others—too many to name, sadly—who are the reason why we care and to whom this book is dedicated.

Elizabeth Reid
Director
HIV and Development Programme
United Nations Development Programme

Introduction

Elizabeth Reid

*Elizabeth Reid is director, HIV and Development
Programme, United Nations Development Programme
(UNDP), New York. Before joining UNDP, she worked
closely with community groups working within the epidemic
in Australia and was responsible for the formulation of
Australia's National HIV/AIDS Strategy. She has extensive
experience in the design and delivery of development
assistance in Asia, the Pacific, the Middle East and Africa.*

The human immunodeficiency virus (HIV) epidemic carries within it forces of destruction and of healing. Which
prevails will be the measure of ourselves and our societies.
It has the power to tear asunder husbands and wives, parents and children; to cause people to turn on one another,
to turn away from one another, to perpetuate acts of indig-
nity and inhumanity. It exacerbates poverty and renders the
rich poor. It subjugates powerful and powerless nations as
well as individuals. Its pain silences. The destructiveness of
its forces is already being felt in affected families and communities as the epidemic unfolds. A refusal to believe, a
resistance of the imagination, and bleakness are all reason-
able responses to these unfurling forces. Personal knowledge
of the epidemic, the experience of its impact, and a fearful
vision of the future create the tone of concern and the sense
of urgency that can be heard in each of these essays.

These forces, and the fallibility of human nature, cause
what Marvellous M. Mhloyi calls a conspiracy of silence. Fears
and feelings remain unaddressed, loved ones become infected,
children are born with no thought for their future. In the

ensuing pain, husbands and wives become estranged, families do not share their sorrow, children live in fear of the unknown. When people are wrapped in this silence, sexuality is expressed in mime, parents do not learn to talk to their children, colleagues are reticent to talk about the future management of their workplace, leaders do not find courage. The destructive forces within the epidemic thrive on secrecy and, as Herbert Daniel says, "public policies that encourage fear, shame, guilt and secrecy [become] the epidemic's accomplices."

An inexorable scenario unfolds after the virus has entered a family or community. Six thousand or more adults become infected every day through an act of love, pleasure or coercion, without being aware that a cataclysm has occurred. Life continues and, unwittingly, these people pass the virus on to others, including their spouses and children. Thus, unlike wars or other significant causes of adult death, whole families are touched: both parents and one or more of their young children become infected. They continue living, unsuspecting, until one of them, often a child, falls ill. The trauma begins with a diagnosis of HIV or acquired immunodeficiency syndrome (AIDS).

Pain is one of the two affective omens of this epidemic. The self-doubt, the anguish and the trauma are relentless. Am I also infected? Am I going to die? Are my parents going to die? Will I be blamed? Will my husband die? What will people say? How dare he? What will happen to my children? What will happen to me? "The first experience of this epidemic," observes Herbert Daniel, "is one of immense moral pain."

People in developing countries usually learn that they are infected when they are already terminally ill. There is little time to put their affairs in order, make their peace with God and loved ones, pass on knowledge and skills to children and coworkers, or plan for the future of their dependents. There is no time to learn to live with the virus.

With the knowledge that their parents are infected or sick, children become insecure and fearful. What will happen to them? Then death robs them of one person they love, then another, then another, leaving them with too much grief to want to go on living. They cannot live with the pain. With the death of both parents, the children often have difficulty staying together and surviving. If they do not have the love and help of others, they become destitute, drifting into the cities, scavenging on the streets, turning to prostitution and banditry to live from day to day.

In a growing number of regions of the world, this is the fate not of a handful of families but of one-tenth of all families—in some communities, one-quarter or more. The fate of nations may soon hang in the balance if the unbearable pain turns to flight, figurative or real, or to brutal slaughter. Glimpses of this future can be seen in these essays: Omari Haruna Kokole's fear for himself and for his sister, Aimée Mwadi's decision not to let her husband place her at risk of infection, Godfrey Sealey's scared and silent friends, the stories from Joan Ross-Frankson's unseen Jamaica, the despair of the young women with whom Ana Vasconcelos works and the grieving families Theresa J. Kaijage counsels.

But the epidemic also has at its centre the power of healing, the lightness of hope, the sound of laughter, and the quality of love. This is its second affective omen, a sign of prophetic significance. It has the capacity to bring out the best in people, as we see in each of these essays. It brings new insights into human nature and interactions. To understand and respond to this epidemic, one must understand daily life and human nature in all their complexities, contradictions, richness and diversity.

It challenges people to want to survive and to want others to do the same. It creates a will to live in both the infected and the uninfected. "I have HIV and I am alive" is Herbert Daniel's celebration of his present and his future. Paradoxically, perhaps, people are empowered by it. They begin to talk to one another, to speak out, to form groups and organizations, to dream a dream of a different life, a different future. They begin to break the silence.

Living within such an epidemic can be a challenging place to be. "We are not a hopeless lot," say Nick Deocampo and Jomar Fleras. "We are a nation of survivors who are resilient in the face of disaster." It is this pervasive quality that justifies the hope, permits the laughter. It is a capacity to cope, an adaptability in times of misfortune.

But it is more than that. It is a transformative power embedded in the imagination that makes possible the sea change from what is to what needs to be. This power takes the silence, the fear, the refusal to acknowledge—all very human responses—and transforms them into the equally human responses of commitment and concern. The imagination introduces a sense of openness to self and others, to the world and to the limitlessness of the future. It loosens the paralysis of silence. Reality is created by the imagination. This mystery of the imagination is a faculty of the soul.

Thus, despite the bleakness of this epidemic, hope springs up again and again wherever people care for one another, wherever love for family and concern for neighbour overcome fear, wherever one person reaches out to help another. This hope is not unrealistic. It is grounded in the discovery of a capacity to cope and a will to live, of compassion and the energy to live it. It is grounded in the imagination and it is the only thing that will carry people through the loss and relentless pain to come. "Hope," says Ian Campbell, "is the basic building block of life."

One of the strongest demands in this book is for an ethical discourse to arise around the epidemic, a demand for moral principles to guide our thinking and our responses—but not an ethic of condemnation, righteousness, or exclusion. Too often the first resort is to isolate or quarantine, to punish or damn, as people struggle with feelings of contamination, disgust or difference. Compassion, caring, togetherness, empathy, community and support are the concepts evoked throughout this collection. "We must tap into traditional cultural values like the spirit of *tulungan*, which fosters concern and participation in any community undertaking. . . . [And into] the spirit of *damayan*, oneness in the community," assert Nick Deocampo and Jomar Fleras. "We must move away from the language of crisis and catastrophe that has permeated the discussion of HIV. We need to develop [a language] that emphasizes hope rather than hopelessness," argues Deborah K. Raditapole. "In the ultimate analysis," says Omari Haruna Kokole, "HIV is our collective disease."

A vocabulary of responsibility, intent, and, where appropriate, murder is demanded. "Countless women who have never had sexual relations with men other than their husbands have become infected as a result of his behaviour." These are the words of Robert E. S. Mugemana, but they are echoed in many of the essays. Legal systems that provide women with little or no recourse to the law or that punish the infected must be reformed. Furthermore, argues Marvellous M. Mhloyi, the inaction of governments must be punished. The development of this ethical discourse must involve churches and faith communities as well as lawyers but must not be left to them. Everyone is implicated and accountable.

The principles being sought are couched not in the traditional ethical vocabulary of rights and justice but rather in ethical concepts such as concern, compassion, oneness, community and solidarity—terms that describe relations between and among people rather than attributes of a particular person. Thus, the pivotal moral concept emerging in these reflections is that of interdependence. "There has never been a time in modern society when human interdependency has been more critical to our survival," reflects Marvellous M. Mhloyi.

Within this ethic of interdependence, of concern and participation, there is a proper place for the language of rights and responsibilities and of justice. Indeed, the absence of this language and these principles in the public arena, particularly in national HIV and AIDS programmes, is lamented throughout the book. For example, Shyamla Nataraj highlights a serious lapse in professional ethics when a medical professional refused to disclose to a woman her HIV status yet readily identified her to a journalist. Marie St. Cyr-Delpe argues that "by failing to make the education of Haitian males the priority, prevention policies essentially absolve men of responsibility while reinforcing the belief that HIV is a woman's disease." Deborah K. Raditapole argues that "this is an issue of human rights, and laws must be changed and new legislation introduced in support of these rights." "I was dying," says Herbert Daniel, "from what I might call a social death, the absence of all human rights."

These concepts of rights and justice need to be embedded in an ethic of mutual support or interdependence. Many forms of interdependence are implicated, and each of them is named in this book. The first is the interdependence of men and women. As so many of these reflections make clear, women alone cannot stop the spread of the virus. Nor can they bear alone the burden of its personal, social, and economic costs. Practices that give witness to women's disempowerment must be changed: wife inheritance, property snatching after the husband's death, infibulation, incest, female infanticide, rape in marriage and elsewhere, dowry, and many others. Men must be involved, and ways must be found to involve them. The problem, Margaret Mwangola counsels, is best approached by sharing rather than confronting. Stories are beginning to be told of relationships between husbands and wives changing, of young women refusing to enter into relationships without guarantees of protection. But these are still rare and isolated incidents. Most women feel unable to protect their lives and those of their children. Unless men and women can forge supportive partnerships of mutual respect and trust, and unless they can share the burdens of sadness and pain, of care and counselling, the epidemic will never be overcome.

The second essential interdependence is between the affected and the not yet directly affected. The infected and those close to them are amongst the most powerful activists and agents of change the epidemic has drawn forth. They give us glimpses of how people can become empowered through trauma and tragedy. Without their voices, people will not be aware of the extent to which the virus has penetrated their families and communities or of its impact on people's lives. The affected provide us with role models, showing communities that they can live without fear, with dignity, within the epidemic. They are helping people understand how to express intimacy, desire and sexuality in the age of the virus. The infected—and they are many—are perhaps the most powerful resource that nations have. Yet they will remain silent and hidden if, in speaking out, they are humiliated, rejected and discriminated against, if they are left alone without support and companionship. There can be no them versus us in the shadow of this epidemic. As Herbert Daniel so eloquently argues, we are all affected, directly or indirectly, for we are all living within it.

The third form of interdependence is between this generation and the next. In its simplest form, this generation owes the next generation the gift of life. For this we created them.

Yet, as Noerine Kaleeba points out, too often it is the men of this generation who are infecting—at times brutally—the girls and young women of the next. We also owe the next generation a life worth living. Thus the silence and shame of this generation must be set aside, as Theresa J. Kaijage indicates, so that parents can talk to their children about being infected and pass on their knowledge and work skills. In return, they must be helped to remain alive as long as possible to nurture and care for their children, and to be nurtured and cared for by them. The next generation will have to give up much to care for and fill in for the missing members of this generation, their parents.

The fourth form of interdependence is between communities and governments. Everywhere the virus spreads, individuals or communities respond. Their responses provide us with hope that the epidemic can be overcome and with inspiration and understanding about how this might come about. But the responsibility to respond cannot be borne by individuals, families, and communities alone. Governments must provide an enabling environment, in particular an appropriate ethical, legal and human rights environment, within which the responses can be sustained. Governments must ensure that the required goods and services—condoms, voluntary counselling, testing services and so on—are accessible and affordable.

Community resources—time volunteered; food, firewood and insights shared; counsel given; transport provided; labour contributed; funds raised; children cared for—lie at the heart of a sustainable response, but these resources must be supplemented. They are not without end and are themselves depleted by the epidemic. They are not usually sufficient. Communities and their organizations know what additional resources they need to be able to continue. They must be empowered to define these resources to others, select them, manage them and account for their use in appropriate ways.

There must be a social contract between community organizations and governments that clearly delineates their respective strengths, rights, and responsibilities and that provides the mechanisms and the means for them to communicate with each other, share their insights and experiences, and work together. This social contract, formal or tacit, must be based on mutual respect and trust. This may not be easy, but it must come about.

The fifth form of interdependence, so often highlighted in these essays, is between and amongst nations. The pattern of spread of the virus—which nations become affected and which individuals are infected and how quickly—is not unrelated to disparities between rich and poor nations and socioeconomic stratification within nations. When will this fact be recognized and acted upon within the world community? The potential for the economic and social devastation of nations inherent within this epidemic is becoming better understood. Certain nations may be brought to the threshold of destitution or destruction. Will the world community respond? Will the world community invest in the psychological support, in education and health and in the technology and technical assistance necessary for these nations to avert such catastrophes? Will there be global social safety nets established to allow nations being rendered dysfunctional by this epidemic to survive?

The closest the world has come to such a safety net is the current system of development assistance. However, this system is fatally flawed for such a purpose; it is inadequate to meet current demands, and its pattern allocation is unrelated to poverty or to the preconditions of human development. Little is invested in education, health or employment creation. If overseas aid is to serve as a global social safety net, it will have to be based on principles of pertinency, adequacy and flexibility. Its first concerns will have to be for human survival and human development, for the creation of a non-exploitative interdependent world.

In all these forms of interdependence, the polarities are between the vulnerable and the powerful, the dominant and the submissive, the centre and the off-centre or marginalized. The distinguishing feature of women, the affected, the next generation, communities and vulnerable nations is their disempowerment, their lack of control over their destinies, their lack of a bargaining position and of collective organization. It is the disequilibrium within which they live. Achieving new forms of partnership, new social contracts between these interdependent groups, will itself require a societal transformation—the transformation of the assumed right to dominate discussion, to speak for, to represent, to control, into new and richer forms of social relations.

The disempowered will have to become articulate, to organize themselves to bargain and negotiate for their rights and, far too often, their lives. It is not that women and young girls do not know what is happening to them and do not fear becoming infected. They are, or feel, powerless to do anything about it. "Who is there to listen to the silent cries of these women and wives? Often their voices go unrecognized within our communities," comments Deborah K. Raditapole. Eka Esu-Williams argues that exploitation, extortion, negative self-perception and societal condemnation ultimately disable many women working in the sex industry. This they share, in one way or another, with most women and young girls, with men who have sex with men, with drug users, and with many others who are affected.

Thus, a precondition for the recognition and establishment of these forms of interdependence is for those affected to come together and remain together. This can be seen in the tragic failure of the men who have sex with men in Godfrey Sealey's Trinidad to break through shame and secrecy to a sense of unity, to come to an understanding that they could be their own best support. Nick Deocampo and Jomar Fleras also observe that activism has been slow to build up in the Philippines among men who have sex with men because they are disorganized and divided by the same class divisions, racism and discrimination found in the heterosexual community. The acknowledgement of the need for those affected to remain together is also evident in Patricia Burke's fears that Jamaica's already frail family struc-ture will unravel, and in the insights that Theresa J. Kaijage's work has given her about the importance of counselling both partners and to link the care of the soon-to-be-parentless chil-dren to the support and care of their parents.

But this coming together, this organization of the vulner-able, must not create boundaries of exclusion or seclusion: who is one of us and who is not. The infected need the space and the time to talk to one another about being infected, but they also need to talk to their spouses and their children. Affected families and their neighbours need to talk. The community of the affected includes everyone. Neither the weak nor the powerful will be able to survive this epidemic alone. If the world is not to be divided, leaders will have to create the con-ditions for people to reach their own decisions rather than having decisions imposed upon them.

The loss and the pain associated with this epidemic are already too much for many to bear. But this too may have a positive aspect, for, as Ian Campbell points out, in every cri-sis there comes a time of helplessness and a need for burden sharing instead of burden bearing. It is a time of truth tell-ing—the end of painful silence and the beginning of close-ness. It creates a basis for togetherness.

Thus talking becomes the basis for healing, the basic strategy for responding to the epidemic. This is borne out elsewhere. For example, when the possibility of talking was created for women who had survived the brutality of the war in Liberia, the act of talking made it possible for them to cry for their loved ones. Giving them food and clothing, they said, made little difference. It was through talking that they regained the will to live. And, as Shyamla Nataraj points out, people want to be able to talk about these things—about not getting infected, about the fear of being infected, about loving and making love to someone who is infected, about the fear of dying. But they do not know how or where.

Truth telling is painful and difficult, however. The retreat into silence is inevitable, more so when sharing brings with it rejection and humiliation and a denial of dignity. This pulling back, of people and of nations, into a silent pain may occur again and again. The talking and the sharing may cease, but the pain and losses will not. They will continue to accumulate until, once again, the burden becomes too much to bear in silence.

The togetherness, the hope, the laughter and the healing of this epidemic are fragile things. They need to be nurtured, safeguarded and encouraged. Shelters will have to be built for them, shelters where, in Ana Vasconcelos' words, people can come together to talk, bathe, rest, eat, dream, think and work out strategies for reaching heaven. And as she has shown in her work, reaching heaven involves a voyage of self-discovery, a voyage toward strength and self-knowledge, a voyage to oneself. It is a voyage of the individual and collective imagination.

1   Racing Against Time

Marvellous M. Mhloyi

*Marvellous M. Mhloyi, Ph.D., is a lecturer at the
University of Zimbabwe. She was a Fulbright/Bernard
Berelson Scholar with the Population Council. Her
research focuses on fertility, family, population policy, and
the psychosocial aspects and determinants of health.*

Although the HIV epidemic has swept the entire world with
incredible speed and devastation, there are significant differences in the prevalence of HIV infection among individual
societies. The world's poorest countries have been the most
severely affected, accounting for approximately 80 per cent
of the global HIV infections. Regional differences are stark,
and in Africa the epidemic is particularly advanced.

The potential impact of HIV can be more clearly assessed
when placed within the proper demographic and socioeconomic context. Because of persistent high levels of fertility
paralleled by declining (but still high) mortality, African
populations are characteristically young, with approximately
45 per cent fifteen years of age and under. Heterosexual sex
is the primary mode of HIV transmission, and because of
the large numbers of women of childbearing age infected
with HIV, perinatal transmission ranks second. Today, these
two modes of transmission account for up to 80 per cent of
HIV infections in Africa.

Because of the inadequacy of death reporting and limited
health facilities, the reported prevalence levels of HIV in

Africa are often underestimated. Nonetheless, given the reported levels, the epidemic's rate of increase, and the demographic profile of many African societies, it is expected that most of sub-Saharan Africa will follow the path of the epidemic observed in central and east African countries.

The Psychosocial Impact of HIV on the Family

When a family member becomes infected with HIV, there are significant disruptions in all aspects of that family's life. Other than being told that the disease is incurable, couples in this situation receive little if any counselling about the possible consequences of infection. What then are the specific effects on a family from the time the first member—usually a child—is diagnosed as HIV-positive to the death of the last adult family member?

Sex is the most common mode of transmission, and the most immediate and frequent response is to assign blame. Often one or both spouses bitterly fault the other's sexual behaviour for their child's illness. The household may be beset by feelings of hopelessness, fear, and isolation. Conflicts arise between the spouses, and children notice the deterioration of their parents' relationship as their sick sibling moves closer to death. Their level of stress and confusion is heightened by charges that their father's behaviour is responsible for their sibling's fatal illness.

Social stigma encourages couples to avoid discussing their situation with outsiders. To a large extent, they may avoid talking to each other. This conspiracy of silence further disrupts family bonds at a time when family members need to share their sorrow. In this atmosphere of strain and silence, children experience fear and uncertainty about the fate of their sibling, their parents' crumbling relationship, and the consequences of the crisis for them.

Couples need to discuss their sexual relationships and the possibility of future pregnancies. Although this is extremely important, it rarely happens. Even under normal circumstances, most people are unwilling to discuss their sexual relations. Some, in the hope of producing a son, may decide on another pregnancy even though the child may be infected. In many instances, contraception is not an obvious or available option. Other couples may practice abstinence, either because the wife is angry and desperately trying to protect her life or because the husband is ashamed, guilty, or afraid of having sex with his infected wife. If the wife chooses to abstain, the couple may divorce and the husband may retain custody of the children. This option, tantamount to divorcing one's children, is untenable to most women. As a result, chances are that the couple will continue an unprotected sexual relationship until the woman conceives again.

Members of the extended family also experience great stress. When a woman becomes ill, in many instances her mother moves into the home to care for her. She may be particularly bitter, blaming her son-in-law for the demise of her grandchild and the terminal illness of her daughter. Although the husband's mother and relatives often live nearby, communication is so severely strained that they feel helpless to assist. Although they too may experience a great sense of loss and sorrow, they do not know how to comfort their son's mother-in-law when their side of the family is held responsible.

This tension sometimes forces the dying woman to return to her family for care, but her relatives may also feel the stress of having to provide for her immediate support as well as the future support of her parentless children. Rarely is there any substantive discussion about how these young children will be cared for. Such conversations are perceived as unwelcome unless raised by the ill mother. The cycle repeats itself when the remaining spouse becomes ill. At the end, the bereaved family is permanently scarred, suffering not only feelings of grief and loss but also a profound sense of social isolation.

What becomes of the children? Having witnessed the deaths of parents and perhaps siblings, their feelings and fears are often unexpressed and unaddressed. Where will they receive the care and nurturing necessary to become productive members of society? It has been shown that foster children generally receive worse treatment than a family's natural-born children. In a discussion on the problem of parentless children in four Ugandan villages particularly hard hit by the epidemic, the thirty guardians participating mentioned food, school fees, health care, and bedding as the most pressing problems. One elderly man noted, "With five children of your own and three orphans to educate, you have to choose."

HIV Intervention Programmes

Most African nations have already instituted national programmes in which HIV education is the dominant feature. Although awareness has been raised, it is poignantly evident that this knowledge has not yet been effectively translated into sustained behaviour and attitudinal change. For example, an ongoing demographic health survey conducted in Zimbabwe recently revealed that among the majority of women who reported having heard of HIV, only a few were doing anything to avoid infection. When asked why, many of them expressed the belief that they were not at risk. The next two most common responses were that they could not avoid AIDS and that they did not know how to avoid AIDS. Obviously, people's knowledge about HIV is incomplete, but in addition to ignorance there is also a high degree of fatalism and denial that crosses age, educational, and regional lines. Equally disturbing was the fact that a significant number of women who knew about HIV believed that people with HIV infection must be quarantined. Although attitudes may have improved since that survey was conducted, the findings underscore the fact that disseminating information effectively enough to change behaviour is of the utmost importance, and this requires time and effort.

When addressing the need to avoid multiple partners, it is crucial to include discussions of polygamy, levirate, and certain other culturally prescribed sexual practices. When changes in traditional practices are called for, information should be provided in a way that helps communities create safe alternatives. Although some may claim that existing programmes already address these issues, evidence strongly suggests that they have been ineffective: the incidence of HIV and other sexually transmitted infections remains high and is increasing in some populations. Governments would prefer to wait for voluntary change, but it is imperative that laws prohibiting these formerly sanctioned cultural practices be instituted and enforced immediately. Such legislation would reduce the helplessness of people who are frightened of breaking ancestral and spiritual tradition but fearful of infection. Granted, these laws would be unpopular, but Africa cannot afford political popularity at the expense of its people's lives.

Programmes promoting the use of condoms must also be accelerated. Africa's pride in parenthood may be the best incentive in any HIV education programme that advocates condom use. The same men who protest condom use may forgo the perceived pleasure of unprotected extramarital sex for healthy surviving offspring.

Education programmes must inform couples of vertical transmission. They need to know that the only way of ensuring that their babies will be born free of HIV infection is for them not to become infected. Making the avoidance of such transmission the basis for safe-sex education can help motivate behaviour change. Such advice would be consistent with local values because it does not counsel against having children.

Couples who are infected with HIV should be advised about the implications of pregnancy. Contraception and abortion should also be discussed, even though these options may be unacceptable or unavailable in cultures where women derive status from maternity. It is important that couples be made aware that their surviving children could become parentless. Parents should be encouraged to consider and plan for alternative caregivers in case they die, and they should prepare their children for such an event.

Women are more vulnerable to HIV because they lack social and economic status and, as a result, have limited decision-making power about issues that affect their welfare and their families. Part of the long-term programme objective should be improving women's socioeconomic condition and addressing the role they often inadvertently play in their own social subjugation. Immediate efforts must be made to empower them with the knowledge and courage needed to encourage and demand safer sex.

To reorder the social system, the men who control it also need empowerment. They must be intellectually and emotionally released from the cultural entrapments that require women to be submissive. Their roles must be redefined to promote the idea that responsible sex, to protect their loved ones and their sexual partners, is an enhancement of manhood. To achieve this, education programmes must overcome their major weakness, which is that they are prescriptive and not based on effective communication.

Existing intervention programmes have also failed to pay sufficient attention to ethical issues. If HIV-infected people were taught that having unprotected sex with an uninfected person is tantamount to murder, some would limit their sexual activities. The use of condoms by a person infected with HIV as a means of minimizing the spread of infection is almost a purely moral consideration. Although messages advocating sexual restraint and monogamy for healthy procreation are more derivative of moral lessons than common education, teaching people about responsible sexual behaviour to protect themselves and others should not be relegated to churches.

It is unfortunate that after thirty years of family planning in Africa, HIV intervention programmes aimed at changing human sexual and reproductive behaviour are repeating the same mistakes. When planning intervention programmes, it is extremely important that members of the targeted population perceive the desired change in behaviour as beneficial to themselves. This was not the case with family planning, which was promoted as a means to curb population growth and was perceived as an invasion. Individuals rarely make fertility decisions based on macro considerations. It is myopic to assume that a scientifically proven problem will be understood by the population. Unless governments and people are convinced, one ends up supplying goods—be they contraceptives for family planning or condoms for HIV prevention—without creating true demand.

It must be stressed that effective communication is the key to cultivating the level of understanding that is needed prior to programme implementation. This goes far beyond using the media; it means dialogue between the interested parties. From dialogue evolves appropriate, community-sensitive education packages, which can be implemented most effectively by trained and experienced personnel who give frank and informed answers.

Counselling programmes for people living with HIV have to be based on local systems. After formulating the counselling strategies, governments should identify at least one person from each of the country's local units and train them to be counsellors. They, in turn, could instruct others, reaching even the smallest communities. It is important that communities designate their own candidates for this training. Some remuneration for the local counsellors should also be given.

Expanding local clinics so that dying people can be cared for by trained health workers should also be considered. This approach would help minimize the risk of spreading infection, release hospital beds to patients suffering from other curable diseases, and allow those diagnosed with AIDS to die peacefully and with dignity.

Increasingly, governments will be faced with the need to provide economic support to the surviving dependents, including children and the aged. Education for parentless children should be available free of charge. Practical and vocational training that has some assurance of economic viability should be considered to help ensure that these youngsters will be able to provide for themselves.

Governments should consider local development projects that employ those residents who are caring for fostered or parentless children. If a bridge is to be constructed, for example, locals would provide paid labour. In Zimbabwe, projects in which local people worked for food during the drought years provided effective assistance while aiding the nation's development.

Coping at the Community Level

At the community level, the extended family assumes responsibility for the care of infirm relatives and children. Grandmothers and older siblings are most likely to care for parentless children. It is important to realize, however, that this obligation may be too daunting for a single individual, given the size of the average African family. For example, a sixty-eight-year-old Ugandan grandmother said in an interview: "I am already weak, and we are poor." HIV had claimed three of her four children, leaving her with one son and twenty-eight grandchildren.

Most extended families need some form of assistance to deal with the burden of HIV. In Tanzania's Kagera district, the community mobilized and established self-help groups to assist parentless children. Residents in Zimbabwe's urban areas formed burial societies, with members contributing funds for funerals. These voluntary societies could be used as models for raising funds to assist children and grandparents.

Coping at the International Level

It is time for African nations to reassess their situations. International organizations have played a vital role in raising awareness and coordinating programmes to challenge the threat of HIV, but most national governments have been dragging their feet. If the world waits for countries to take serious action, it may be too late. In this decade, we must adopt a more aggressive approach. Individuals, communities, national governments, and international organizations each have a key role to play in addressing the problem. The challenge is how each fits into the puzzle to produce the greatest impact.

No international organization has a wide enough latitude to push governments to act. This gap might be filled by a neutral international coalition with enough experts from each continent to form subgroups. These experts would include researchers, policymakers, programme designers, and implementers drawn from existing regional networks to facilitate communication between the group and the regions. Their most important mission would be to develop and implement a more effective and efficient mechanism for pushing nations to act immediately. They would also serve as brokers between countries and donor agencies, assisting in defining and prioritizing problems and identifying the type of aid needed.

The HIV epidemic clearly makes demands that are far beyond the economic capacity of most African countries. Thus, cooperation from the international community will be needed. However, it is of major importance that African countries find an African solution to this problem. This process has been initiated through intergovernmental cooperation at the highest ministerial level and has been addressed by the recent Organization of African Unity (OAU) declaration. By forming networks, countries could inform one another about the levels and trends of HIV infection among their populations, the nature and types of programmes effectively initiated, mistakes made, and the problems that remain unresolved. In the absence of outsiders, this could facilitate more open communication among African nations. This step would assist every country regardless of the epidemic's impact on it. It would also assist in the creation and development of intervention programmes, thereby saving time and resources.

Networks have already begun forming in many regions. The African regional network of AIDS service organizations (AFRICASO) has subregional affiliates in southern, western, and northern Africa and focal points working toward the creation of subregional networks in central and eastern Africa.

African countries should also initiate fund-raising to assist in the implementation of their HIV programmes. These initiatives should build on the interdependency of African countries. For example, there is an urgent need to prevent the epidemic from exacerbating the already dire refugee problem. Identifying and prioritizing national as well as regional needs could assist donor agencies in their funding assessments.

Africa's national governments are the most important players in this life-or-death drama. Most central and some southern African countries are already beyond the first stages. These countries must invest their resources in three key areas: improving educational and counselling strategies, designing home-based care for the growing number of patients, and preparing for the care and support of the increasing population of parentless children.

The dominant theme of these strategies must be the effect of HIV on everyone's life. There has never been a time in modern history when human interdependency has been more critical to our survival. The degree to which this message is communicated will determine the level of commitment to combating this problem and the mobilization of funds and resources.

Investing in the Future

Though these recommendations are expensive, the expense is relative. Countries must consider the potential impact of

HIV on their economies: the loss of productive and trained personnel, the cost of replacing them, the erosion of the tax base, the difficulty of motivating parentless children to rebuild and become productive citizens. This assessment should be weighed against the cost of an effective intervention programme. Nations can reorder priorities to make the necessary budgetary changes. This more efficient management of internal funds could finance the most urgent components of HIV programmes. Political leaders who fully appreciate the problem the epidemic poses can effect significant changes with minimal financial input if they are truly committed. The gap between the estimated total costs and what countries can afford will require international assistance, which is most effective when it complements the internal crusade.

The radical change imposed by HIV is too rapid and too extensive to have anything but the most dire psychosocial, demographic, and economic impact on most, if not all, sub-Saharan countries. The loss of so many productive members of society increases the dependency ratio and will undoubtedly affect already stagnant or diminishing economic growth rates. African governments must realize that if the epidemic continues unabated, all investments currently made in every sector of their economies will be undermined.

This epidemic is devastating the African continent with each passing moment. It will not be the same world if half or more of the next middle-aged generation in Africa is composed of parentless children. The next generation will condemn us for patting one another on the back, comfortable with a few success stories, while refraining from taking the radical steps necessary to reduce and stop the spread of this disease.

As I write, I feel strongly that this is not the best way for me to exert the most influence on this epidemic. Even if I had the most wonderful ideas and solutions, great damage would have been done by the time this book reached you. This epidemic is without precedent in the modern world and demands action rather than writing. We need constructive action by individuals, communities, nations, and international organizations. Our biggest challenges are to avoid complacency, overcome denial, and create a network of assistance built on dialogue, sincerity, trust, respect, and responsibility. Even the worst epidemics of the past failed to make the human race extinct, and with that ray of hope, nations must be encouraged to forge ahead.

2 One More Risk in a Very Risky World

Ana Vasconcelos

Ana Vasconcelos has been working to promote the welfare of, and to minimize the spread of HIV among, the children and adolescents who work and live in the streets and brothels of Recife, Brazil. To reach the girls of the street, Vasconcelos has created a network of educational, medical, and shelter services anchored by Casa de Passagem (Passage House), located in the heart of downtown Recife.

interviewed by Edison Maciel

Edison Maciel is a Brazilian journalist and photographer who travels extensively throughout South America covering the region for the Danish newspaper Information.

Whenever a worker loses his job, his children head for the streets because they have a better chance of bringing home what the family needs to survive. A man begging is of little use, but a child begging can always bring in some money. So the economic factor is of primary importance when sending one's children to the streets. Up to 30,000 children a day take to the streets of Recife, Brazil, seeking money to help their families survive. About 4,000 of these youngsters exist entirely within a street culture.

In 1987, I helped found the Task Force on Children and, in 1988, SOS Children, the first group concerned with providing legal assistance to children in the city of Recife. Besides being an attorney, I have completed postgraduate work in urban and rural development. I was practicing law when my cousin Jarbas Vasconcelos was elected prefect of Recife. Because I admired him a great deal, I accepted when he asked me to assume responsibility for city policy relating to the welfare of street children. I began as vice president of the Special Legion of Recife, a nongovernmental agency, and was also responsible for advising the prefect on labour issues and social affairs. I was trying to coordinate the activities of the prefecture and the Special Legion of Recife in order to get people to take an integrated approach to the problem of street children rather than formulating policy in isolation.

In 1987, we began distributing condoms to all children who asked for them irrespective of age. Based on feedback we got from other institutions, we realized that there was major discrimination against commercial sex workers and street girls. People began to be more disgusted and repulsed by the girls. Culturally, any woman in the streets is considered a commercial sex worker, even if she is not. Because she is living in the streets, she is a symbol of the ugliness of the sex trade industry and sin. Above and beyond this, the girls came to represent the danger of HIV.

From 1986 to 1987, I had been trying to ensure that street girls received the same attention as the boys. I had thirty-five specialists working with me—thirty-three women and two men. These women had problems working with the girls because, as they told me, "Girls are elusive, they slip through your fingers. It is as if they do not want anything, as if they actually like both sex work and the streets."

I knew that this was not true. Beginning in June 1988, I went out into the streets in earnest. I would work in the office until early afternoon and then go out to meet the girls. As a result, I began to understand the problems my coworkers were experiencing while working with the girls. If you try to work with children only in terms of employment and political organization, you will get nowhere, because these children are never going to earn more than a pittance. People who have a political view fail to ask, Who is this child? What is she feeling and thinking? What does she want? What makes her tick?

People who are concerned about the girls themselves find that they have specific problems they want to discuss: sexuality, what it means to be a girl and to be out in the street; what it is to experience pregnancy, an abortion, menstruation. Girls also want to discuss sexual violence. A girl will say, "I did not die, but I was raped. I paid with my body, with my very life." They want to talk about how boys boss them in the streets and beat them up. These girls are completely hemmed in, and they want to talk about these issues.

In certain respects, the boys take from society, whereas the girls who get into commercial sex work support our society. In fact, sex work helps keep many families together, because men have a double standard: a wife at home and a sex worker in the streets. In truth, girls do not upset the system. They play an important role, which is to satisfy men. They do not challenge the system, although some girls do get into stealing. The boys disrupt and steal and get into many more confrontations with the police.

Girls follow a pattern that we are studying. When a girl leaves home, she tries to succeed as a peddler, but she has to compete in the male-dominated labour market. A girl might dress like a boy to wash cars. When the boys discover that she is a girl, they send her packing because the street turf is all divided up. As in real life and in society at large, the girls have no place that is theirs. Girls have no place in the labour market of the streets, so they fall in with gangs. They fight to be able to go on peddling; some succeed, but others do not. They end up in sex work or dead. Girls have no choice in the matter because violence is the way of the streets. They will be raped constantly. The only escape is to sell their bodies in order to obtain a little peace. Sometimes sex work is a form of self-defence. As the girls say, "We are going to sell what they want to take by force or by charm."

As a rule, all the girls say, "I have to help my mother." And in fact, they do help—even those whose mothers have thrown them out. I think that every girl who has a family has the desire to help out. They even say, "You feel bad about eating when you know your mother is not eating." This concern is always present. Almost all the girls have some contact with their families, even if it is only once a year at Christmas. All of them have memories of their families, although some have no families left because of death.

When I talked with girls in the streets to see how we could carry out our work in mutual respect, they would tell me to get the hell out of there, because they knew that I was the vice president of an institution. They would ask me, "Don't you know that this is the way to hell here?" This made quite an impression on me. For the girls, the very culture of the streets was the road to hell. Then I saw that some Protestant religious groups were telling them that everybody on the street was going to hell, because the only ones there were crazy people, thieves, and drug addicts. So there was a need to create a special place where people could find a way to heaven.

That was the origin of the idea of a house—a temporary shelter—where people could talk, bathe, eat, and work out strategies for getting to heaven. This heaven was a beautiful place because it was reached through a voyage of self-discovery, the idea of being oneself, discussing one's problems, getting to know oneself. That was the heaven that people were thinking of, that I was thinking of, for the girls—the heaven of truth.

On 15 May 1989, we succeeded, with the help of some friends, in opening a temporary shelter. Today we have two shelters and various houses where we assist an average of 100 girls a day. Others we see on the run, so to speak; they pass by, pick up a condom, get some information, and go to one of our doctors. When they find out that they have contracted HIV, there is great despair. That is when they seek us out. They arrive crying that they have AIDS; they are afraid that they are going to die.

We are a small group, only twenty-five technical specialists, but we provide the lead. Half of our concerns are with bare survival, so we realize that our project cannot reach very many people. Our staff has their work cut out for them every day. We just completed a two-month street campaign in which we distributed 16,000 condoms.

In this environment, the incidence of sexually transmitted infections is incredible. Doctors cannot believe what they are seeing. Ten-year-old girls have diseases that, in the past, only thirty-year-olds would have. There are even moments when I think that I have HIV. We take care of girls who come in to us bleeding, who have been raped or stabbed. Sometimes we have gloves, sometimes we do not. Sometimes I have the feeling that we are all infected. I think we need a greater sense of solidarity with respect to HIV and AIDS in this country.

Approximately 10 per cent of our girls are infected with HIV, but this is only a rough estimate. We have already lost two girls with whom we used to work every day to AIDS. There are times when you think that this disease is going to affect everybody. You know that a particular boy does not have any of the symptoms yet, but he has tested positive. That boy is having sex with who knows how many people. So when is it going to show up?

We supply condoms to the girls, and they are glad to get them because they are expensive to buy. On a single night, we took 1,000 condoms to distribute in the streets and our supply was exhausted. Some customers carry condoms—

middle-class people or foreigners. Some girls are even refusing customers if no condom is used. So customers are beginning to realize that they lose nothing by using condoms.

It is a challenge to the machismo of those customers who react negatively: "Do you think I am sick? Do you think you are better than me? How can you, a prostitute, think that you are better than me?" But the girls respond, "It's not because I am better than you, but because I can have a disease too, and might infect you." Our people have put a great deal of effort into helping the girls with these dialogues. Some girls play the role of customers and others play themselves. This role-playing has yielded positive results.

We also have three theater groups, each one made up of seven girls; they perform in the streets and even in the brothels. They put on a play entitled "It's AIDS," saying that A is for *amor* (love), I for *informaçao* (information), D for *dignidade* (dignity), and S for *saude* (health). The play is about a woman and her daughters who are suddenly left without any means of support. In desperation, the woman opens a brothel and begins to make money, but she does not pay any attention to HIV. Ultimately, only the mother and two of her daughters survive. In the end, the mother understands that if the brothel is to continue and if she is to continue to make money, the brothel must be clean and well-organized, and the question of HIV and AIDS must be discussed.

People are spreading the word. I have no doubt that this is thanks to the energy of the girls—a very powerful energy. These girls are strong. They know that they are going to die before they reach the age of twenty-five, yet they continue to live life. I think that they are miracles. We have another group of girls called health protection outreach workers. Each year we train about thirty of them, and they pass on information to other girls. This is methodical work that requires patience and reliance on one another. I believe that we have changed behaviours and made a substantial contribution.

This city and the rest of the country are a joke. I open the morning newspaper and I read that the state is unable to spend any more money on HIV; it says that there is no money in the budget to care for people with HIV. Even the funds to pay the staff have run out. Moreover, condoms are not being distributed in this city. Often, the condoms are held up in the health department because there are certain prescribed procedures for distributing them. In my opinion, there should be a condom dispenser on every street corner of this city. They say that the population is becoming depraved. So be it. But think of the difference between distributing condoms and treating the entire population for HIV. Isn't it much cheaper to distribute condoms?

I believe that there is no money because it is earmarked for other purposes. There is much more concern today about industrialization than about saving people who are dying. I do not dispute that we have to become a country that is able to compete in the world market, but I also believe that we must rescue this population. What is happening is that 10 per cent are going forward and 90 per cent are dying along the way.

Society approaches commercial sex workers and homosexuals as if they pose a threat to society. Obviously the prejudices are very strong and people are very afraid, including health and social workers. People's fear of intimacy has increased. As a general rule, the government's campaigns are designed to frighten people even more: "Watch out, AIDS is going to get you." "AIDS kills." When a campaign is so heavy-handed and does not suggest any alternatives, at a certain point, people do not pay attention anymore. A girl living in the slums without enough money to survive is not going to become sexually inactive. The only pleasure left for the poor is sex. They have no other outlets; they cannot indulge in fantasy by going to a shopping mall to buy nice clothes.

In the final analysis, HIV is just one more risk in a very risky world. As they say, "AIDS has no name in Brazilian! So I am going to worry about a disease that has a Brazilian name," like venereal disease, hunger, and malnutrition. What we need is not a campaign that says that AIDS is going to get you, but one that says, "We have ways to help you avoid getting sick."

What are we going to do with people, exterminate them? Isn't HIV a form of extermination? We need a population that is much more aware. I have been thinking lately that what we need is people who are demanding. How can we get the people to demand more? I believe that the president and other government officials would create new policies if the people were organized, but our people have lost their bearings. Why is this? Because 70 per cent are hungry.

At forty-six years of age, I am very tired because I have been working in the streets for six years without rest. There are moments when I say, "My God, I think I'm going to kick the bucket this year." I am travelling a great deal. I will be going to Maceio and Fortaleza soon. I am also involved with the women's movement, and I see that feminist groups are beginning to be concerned about the girls on the street. This is a good thing. These people want to hear about the experiences of others and want to set up programmes similar to ours. There are no other programmes specifically targeted to street girls.

We get some government funding, but we need help that is more sustained. The shelter is not the only programme that needs more systematic help; all the groups need it. How can we work if funding is not provided on a planned basis? So we survive, in these enormous vacuums, with outside funding. We get money from Germany, from the Netherlands, and a little from the United States. Our heartfelt thanks go to all the people at these international agencies: Terre des Hommes, Caritas, Bread for the World, Miserium, and others. Many of them are Catholic agencies that give us money, respect us, and do not put any pressure on us. There are the Dutch agencies such as Norbe, Kinder, and the Altiplano Alternative, and an American agency called the Catholic Children's Foundation; there are also private organizations such as Humankind and Childhope in England. Occasionally we receive a small grant from UNICEF.

I would like to thank my staff for all their support; these people exist only to help others. We are stronger for their efforts. I want to set up hundreds of shelters in this country and abroad. A shelter, as the name implies, is a place where you can seek information and support and get the strength you need to go on living life, to be respected, to rest, to think. I want people to raise children in harmony with the environment, in harmony with nature; to educate them and to save them from extermination at the hands of HIV.

3   In the Epidemic's Shadow

Shyamla Nataraj

> *Shyamla Nataraj started the South India AIDS Action*
> *Programme in 1991. A former newspaper editor, she*
> *currently works as a freelance journalist. After report-*
> *ing on the detainment of HIV-positive commercial*
> *sex workers in Madras, she helped bring their*
> *case before the court, which led to their release.*

"White man's balloons. That's what we call condoms here,"
Selvi splutters, as smothered giggles erupt into general laughter among the women gathered on the floor of her house. Selvi,
who lives in one of Madras' slums, is barely nineteen and
already big with her third child. "I'll have an operation after
this one. No balloons for me, thank you."

Fatima nods vigorously, saying, "I had to go and get mine
done without my in-laws knowing about it. Thank God I did,
a fifth kid would have been impossible."

Gowri, one of the few among the group who still has not
had an operation, explains, "The doctor said I was too weak,
no blood you know. So I have to wait."

Lakshmi, with a sly grin, asks, "But that doesn't stop your
husband, does it?"

Amid blushes, Gowri plaintively says, "I hope I don't get
pregnant again, but what can I do?"

"Lakshmi, you're just the right person to talk about all this.
Tell us, have you ever used a condom?"

While steadily chewing a wad of tobacco, Lakshmi replies,
"You mean white man's balloons? Well, we actually used it

once, but my man didn't like it at all. I remember him complaining about having to throw it out in the street. You know how these kids pick them up and play with them."

"The children blow them up or fill them with water and play around. God, they can hold an awful lot of water," her friend Gowri quips mischievously. Patting her suckling infant, she says, "When I had this child here, the nurse at the government hospital thrust a handful of them at me and told me to ask my husband to use them. He was livid. He yelled, 'You want to castrate me, woman,' and flung the whole lot out of the house."

"Mine would immediately think I was seeing another man," says Fatima, whose husband keeps another wife somewhere else in the city. "These men are so suspicious. 'Where are you going?' 'What are you doing there?' 'Who are you talking to?' Imagine asking them to use condoms!"

In India, it is not just the Gowris and Selvis who face the problem of unwanted pregnancies and carry the responsibility for avoiding them. The lack of birth control unites all women. With India's population at 880 million and expected to total more than 1 billion by the year 2000, the need for an aggressive family-planning effort has never been greater. Yet the government-initiated family-planning campaign has focused solely on women. As Dr. Mira Shiva reported in an article in *Health for Millions*: "Even when vasectomies on the male are easier to perform and cause less complications, they are unpopular, mainly because they are associated with impotence. No attempts have been made to dispel this myth while great efforts have been made to convince women to get sterilized as the only solution inherent in the social structure."

The spread of HIV is now prompting government and private organizations alike to take a fresh look at existing policy. Successful social marketing of condoms by Population Services

International India, a nonprofit society committed to family welfare located in New Delhi, has led to a belated recognition of the need for effective condom marketing strategies.

The need to reach and educate the populace is acute. For example, women who work in the commercial sex trade say that clients rarely, if ever, use condoms. And many of the women themselves are unaware of the fact that condom use can prevent sexually transmitted infections (STIs). As one woman said, "I thought they were only for family planning. But I'm careful. I can make out if somebody has something by looking at him, his nose, his hands, his ears."

Commercial condom manufacturers still resist associating their product with STIs, HIV, or AIDS. They prefer to position their product as upmarket and trendy. Although this male-focused marketing strategy has increased sales, consumers continue to be from the upper-income brackets, while the man on the street remains unconvinced. For him, the decision to use a condom has to transcend more than his psychological resistance. It must be viewed in the context of his physical environment, the way he lives, the facilities he lacks, and the lifestyle imposed on him by his surroundings.

Muthu's attitude is fairly typical: "I work in the port, coolie work. Sometimes there is too much heat in my body from working so many hours in the sun so I have to cool off. So I have a drink with some friends, watch a movie, eat some mutton curry, and have fun with a woman. So do many of my friends. No, we don't use condoms, that's for family planning. Besides, when the chance comes who'll go looking for them? And why pay so much if you can't get the same jolly? Once, in the beginning, I got a venereal disease but I took some medicine and it was all right. Now I'm careful to see what kind of girl I pick up. I can make out who's safe by seeing her face."

"Condoms?" snorted Perumal derisively. "What for? My wife has already got operated on so we don't need any family planning. These health people keep handing them out to us, but we give them to the kids or throw them away. I can't imagine anybody using them. Besides, where would they get rid of them afterwards?"

Perumal's living conditions make his concern about disposal all too understandable. He, his wife, and their three growing children share approximately 100 square feet of space with his two brothers. Their home is one of 700 in a colony meant for no more than 300. The tightly squeezed houses back onto narrow lanes that separate one row from another. Although the lanes and houses are kept scrupulously clean, the common areas around the few water taps and the block of toilets are filthy. This is due partly to overcrowding and partly to an erratic water supply and no system of garbage disposal.

Despite the terrible overcrowding and poor sanitation, Perumal is resigned, even content. "If I were back in my village, I would live in a cleaner place but would have no income. Here at least I make enough to feed my family and to send my kids to school. What else can I do?" Most of the men in the colony work as rickshaw pullers, day labourers, or construction workers. To supplement their incomes, some of the men used to sell their blood to the hospitals, but they are not buying now. According to Perumal, "We go to small private places where nobody makes a fuss."

Perumal's home is located in one of the thousands of slums that dot the city of Madras and house hundreds of thousands of people. Each day, migrants come to the city in search of employment, and new colonies appear. This housing phenomenon is occurring in all of India's cities as runaway population growth and increasing poverty destroy the environment and set into motion huge streams of distress migration.

It is estimated that there will be an increase in the nation's urban population of 100 million by the year 2001. Only 60 million of this increase will be due to natural growth. Migration is the major reason for most of this population growth. Agriculture is the principal activity among 75 per cent of the population in rural India, and when drought occurs, people are forced to seek alternative employment. The paucity of labour-intensive industries in rural areas, a lack of alternative skills-training facilities, and the concentration of wealth in urban centres forces people like Perumal out of their traditional niches and into the cities. It is rare that these migrants ever return to their villages. As Perumal's sturdy twelve-year-old son put it: "Agriculture is for illiterates. I want a government job."

"Unemployment is our biggest problem," observed Lakshmi the next time we spoke. "Men can always find jobs as construction workers or coolies at the docks, but it's bloody hard work. No wonder the men drink so much. But after a while they can't do without the stuff. Then they lose their jobs, and it's up to the women again to feed the family. I know some women who buy their husbands their liquor so they can keep an eye on how much he drinks. Besides, if he is at home, there's not much chance of him whoring around.

"But women aren't saints either. I suppose it's all natural. What else is there to do? I had a lover myself before I married this man. My first child is actually his. Everybody knows, but so what? It's really no big deal. There are a lot of girls in this colony who aren't married but have kids. How do you think they look after them? Certainly not by selling sweets," she winked knowingly. "There are even some men here who like men, you know what I mean? And many of them are married. Some wives know, others don't, but what can they do?"

The emergence of HIV in India has focused attention on certain behaviours that were considered foreign and impossible in our country. "Come with me one night and I'll show you at least three respectably married, well-known men trying to make contact," challenges Ashok Row Kavi, the Bombay-based publisher of India's first magazine for homosexuals. The existence of homosexuality is finally being acknowledged, as is the fact that premarital sex is on the rise. Several studies at government-run abortion clinics around the country have found increasing rates of premarital pregnancy. Another survey revealed a significant presence of STIs among unmarried girls in a rural area in the state of Maharastra.

In addition to disproving the smug assumption that India's superior value system could prevent the spread of HIV, the Maharastra survey clearly indicates our vulnerability. The high incidence of STIs is now acknowledged as a factor that enables the spread of HIV. A UNICEF-sponsored nationwide survey found that one out of every twenty Indian men and women suffers from some form of STI. The lack of sex education, the reluctance to discuss sex and related matters openly, the stigma attached to sexual issues, and the prevailing belief in folk remedies cause people to delay seeking treatment, thus facilitating the spread of HIV. Despite the presence of more than 300 STI clinics throughout the country, medical treatment is sought only as a last resort.

The superior attitudes adopted by doctors at clinics, where educational material and prevention information are conspicuously absent, only perpetuate people's ignorance of the epidemic. The dearth of trained female specialists also discourages women from seeking treatment for STIs. Amid rising concern about HIV, many nongovernmental organizations (NGOs) are beginning to recognize the need to address the prevalence of STIs within communities. Despite reservations about discussing sex and individual behaviour, one social worker who works with male clients says, "Discussing sex is really not as difficult as it is made out to be. People want to be able to talk about some of these things, only they don't know how and where." Another social worker who works with women in the slums of Madras agrees: "It's amazing how frank these people are. But that can happen only if you can also be frank about yourself. I feel that takes more time and effort."

Women who work in the commercial sex industry are also vulnerable to contracting HIV. Vijaya has been a commercial sex worker for more than ten years. In 1986, when surveillance had just begun, she was one of the first women who tested positive for HIV infection. When questioned about HIV, she retorts, "What AIDS? I don't have anything, no fever, no diarrhoea. See my hands and legs. I'm perfectly normal." Vijaya was one of 500 women arrested in 1989 under the Prevention of Immoral Traffic Act. She was detained after the expiration of her sentence because of her seropositivity. In late 1990, after the Madras High Court's precedent-setting ruling that HIV-related detention was illegal, Vijaya and other commercial sex workers were released and have returned to work. In an uncharacteristically confiding mood, she once said, "You say I'm infected and that I can spread the virus to a man. But what can I do if he refuses to use a condom? If I insist, he'll go to somebody else, and I have a living to make. I want to see that my son is educated and has a good job. If somebody can assure me of that and promise me a roof over my head with a decent income, I'll stop this work. But until then, what's the use of all this talk? I'll just carry on. What else can I do?" It's ironic that female commercial sex workers are seen as the source of infection, when they have been infected by male clients.

One positive outcome of the Madras High Court ruling has been the shift in policy from eliminating commercial sex work to providing support to those who engage in it to make a living. Surveys to determine the women's priorities are being conducted for the first time. Predictably, their own health is far down on the list. Their main concern is about their children, followed by a demand that the police be kept off their backs. To its credit, the government is listening, and several states have ordered the police to lay off. In another major development, male clients are now being targeted for health education as well. Organizations are exploring the possibility of taking STI and HIV education door-to-door in the red-light areas. The rationale is that all people should be treated as human beings who are vulnerable when practicing unsafe sexual behaviour rather than as specific groups that get labelled as pools of infection. Perhaps the best thing that has occurred is that women are beginning to demand recognition. As a result, the country's first union of commercial sex workers has been established.

Drug use is also not as uncommon as generally thought. According to Shanti Ranganathan, director of the T. T. Ranganathan Clinical Research Foundation, a well-known detoxification centre for substance abuse in Madras, "We're seeing more drug addicts than before. Those who are addicted cut across all classes. We have executives, businessmen, students, slum people. More men than women of course, but more women than earlier. We didn't have any injecting drug users until a couple of years ago, so it's obvious this is catching on."

In an effort to address this relatively new aspect of the epidemic, voluntary groups are working in collaboration with government to explore the possibility of setting up needle-exchange centres in several parts of the country. In a radical departure from the norm, most authorities are willing to try anything that works without getting drawn into controversies. *Nonjudgmental, voluntary, anonymous, confidential,* and *counselling* are the new buzzwords that sit with surprising comfort on the bureaucratic tongue. This has, without a doubt, helped heal some of the traditional distrust that inevitably exists between activists and government.

Problems still remain, however. One is the absence of a policy that mandates informing infected people of their status. Another is the persistent disregard for patient confidentiality. Shantini holds an executive position in a corporation. She is married and is the mother of two small children. She is also HIV-positive. Her status was discovered the last time she donated blood, but she has yet to be informed. Talking to her, I find it impossible to believe that this beautiful, articulate, and obviously intelligent woman should not know something that will affect her life so drastically. "What do we do after we tell her she is seropositive? We just don't have the facilities for pre- and post-test counselling," explains one doctor, nor are any support services available. Yet the doctor showed no compunction in disclosing her status to me, which points out a serious lapse in professional ethics.

The reluctance of medical personnel to treat HIV-positive patients is another problem. Veenet and Rohit Oberoi are brothers with haemophilia who became infected though the use of blood products. Once it was known that they were HIV-positive, Veenet says, "all the hospitals in the area refused to treat us." In addition to being refused medical help, the brothers, who live with their parents in a flat in New Delhi, have been shunned by their neighbours.

Screening of blood and blood products is now mandatory, and a network of sixty-seven surveillance centres has been established. But the lackadaisical approach to hospital hygiene and the fact that people like Perumal continue to sell blood to private clinics—where screening may not be strictly adhered to—are causes for concern. The possibility of cross infections occurring in hospitals cannot be ruled out. Money is also an issue here: less than 1 per cent of the total federal budget goes to public health. Medical staff constantly face shortages of items ranging from disposable needles and gloves to major equipment such as incinerators.

Unfortunately, mudslinging and manipulation are going on, as is usually the case when large sums of money are involved. The prospect of trips abroad, exposure at international meetings, and professional recognition has set off a tug-of-war among medical specialists over who should be acknowledged as HIV authorities. This attitude is also increasingly evident among NGOs, which must compete with one another for the limited funds available for HIV programmes on both national and international levels. Other organizations are quick to resent the attention being paid to HIV and AIDS, and they accuse those involved of jumping on the bandwagon.

Yet HIV offers the best chance for India to examine policy issues that have not been debated so far. The government has taken a fresh look at the AIDS prevention bill that was introduced in 1989. At that time, several organizations denounced it as discriminatory against infected people and a violation of civil liberties. The bill allowed for involuntary detention of HIV-positive people. It has now been reviewed by a select committee, which will discuss, among other things, licensing commercial sex work, maintaining patient confidentiality, and providing support services for patients and their families.

As one person put it, "The best thing about HIV is that I can peg it to almost anything: public health, accountability, rational drug policy, sex education, sexuality, and gender issues. Then people will start listening." The good news is that some already have.

4   Struggling with Contradictions

Nick Deocampo and Jomar Fleras

> *Nick Deocampo is a filmmaker and the director
> of the Mowelfund Film Institute. Jomar Fleras
> is a playwright and HIV activist.*

As the Philippine night descends, much of the façade that masks this predominantly Catholic society is stripped away to reveal Manila's stark realities. The glow of the capital city's neon-lit streets reveals a netherworld where the commercial sex industry thrives.

Elmer is but one among many who make their living there. His regular source of income comes from stagings of *toro*, the local lingo for anal or vaginal sexual intercourse performed in public. First popularized in underground heterosexual bars during the 1960s, *toro* has found its way to those gay bars known for masturbation contests and sex orgies. Elmer, who takes the receptor role, is one of the district's best-known performers. Lured into the sex trade at an early age, he has performed this act nightly before a jeering crowd for the last ten years. It is an ugly, dehumanizing way of making a living, but with the money, Elmer, who lives in the slum colony of Tondo, supports a son, an ailing grandmother, a number of brothers, and several other relatives.

He has heard of HIV and knows that it kills. He is concerned because it threatens not only his life but also the lives of those who depend on him for support. Yet Elmer has only a vague idea of how HIV is transmitted and how infection can be prevented. This degree of ignorance about the disease remains alarmingly high throughout the country. The distortion and confusion that surround the subject have created a climate in which people affected by and at risk of contracting the disease demonstrate complex and conflicting responses: anxiety, fear, guilt, apathy, denial, anger, and fatalism.

Perhaps to deflect the fear, perhaps in denial, Elmer has adopted a to-hell-with-it attitude that borders on hysteria. He violently objects to having an HIV blood test and does not use or request the use of condoms during his shows. When asked what he would do if he became HIV-positive, Elmer candidly replies, "I will get a can of gasoline and set myself on fire," noting that it would be front-page news. Elmer's reaction, though histrionic, is not an isolated phenomenon. In a recent survey, 28 per cent of male sexual workers said that they would commit suicide if they became infected with HIV.

Here in the Philippines, to understand reality one must struggle with contradictions. Our colonial history can best be described as 300 years of convent life under Roman Catholic Spain and forty years of Hollywood under the United States. We have undergone a barrage of indoctrinations from two extreme ideologies—the medieval spirituality of the Catholic Church and the modernity and commercialism of American pop culture. America's teaching of sexual freedom has helped foster behaviours that enable the spread of HIV in the Philippines. The Catholic faith, as bequeathed by Spanish friars, has instilled reactionary religious beliefs that also help the disease's spread.

This social history has resulted in a double standard and is responsible for many of the contradictions that pervade Filipino life. These contradictions manifest and represent a distinct aspect of the national personality. Youngsters are torn between the family's strict moral codes and peer pressure to break sexual taboos. As a rite of passage, groups of friends commonly arrange for boys to lose their virginity in brothels. Marriage is extolled as the social ideal, yet married men regularly seek extramarital sex. Sex work is regularly denounced and blamed on the American military and other foreigners. Yet in one study, female sex workers said that 75 per cent of their clients were local married men. On paydays, it is common to see Filipino men trooping to massage parlours, which are fronts for the commercial sex industry.

These contradictions are also illustrated in the ways some people seek to reconcile their sense of powerlessness with the divine. In the very heart of Ermita, Manila's red-light district, is a church where sex workers pray before plying their trade. Images and icons of saints meant to inspire luck can also be found in brothels. Many commercial sex workers wear religious scapulars, crosses, or amulets as protection against sexually transmitted infections. It is not unusual to find Filipinos employing a combination of folk Catholicism, mysticism, and superstition in dealing with HIV. Adhering to the belief that everything is the work of divine Providence, that all is a matter of fate, creates a sense of helplessness and insecurity in many Filipinos.

One shudders to think how easily HIV can become a crisis in Manila. The city has more than 1,000 bars, massage parlours, and discos catering to sex-seeking tourists. During Ferdinand Marcos' regime, sex tours were in high demand, and commercial sex work claimed not only women and men but children as well. The permissive sexual climate during that twenty-year period was merely symptomatic of the decay in the country's economic, political, and moral structure—a decay epitomized by political repression and the conspicuous consumption of our conjugal dictators Ferdinand and Imelda Marcos.

Today the economy of the Philippines is devastated. Seventy per cent of the population lives in poverty. Although our literacy rate is one of the highest in Asia, the quality of education leaves much to be desired. People are ignorant about basic health issues, and the commercial sex industry runs at full tilt.

We are tired of fighting powerful tyrants and colonial masters; tired of typhoons, earthquakes, floods, and other natural calamities; tired of the poverty, corruption, and political instability that have gripped our nation for generations. To many Filipinos, the threat of HIV, with its insidious power to spread undetected, is another fearsome and fatiguing burden.

The advent of HIV was met with the customary denial and suppression of information. The United States and those politicians with close ties to it were blamed for the virus' incursions. Opposition leaders used the issue to criticize the government for advocating sex-related tourism, and the media sensationalized the disease by focusing on its incurable nature.

To counter the fear, jokes about HIV and AIDS abounded. The government's report of only 218 cases of HIV infection at the end of 1990 led many Filipinos to believe that the situation was not serious. The public does not realize that if we do not intervene now, we will have a serious problem in the near future.

The last decade has witnessed a substantial rise in migration. More than 1 million Filipinos have left home seeking temporary work abroad. There is little doubt that some returning workers are infected with the virus.

The U.S. military presence in our country has always been associated with commercial sex work and consequently with sexually transmitted infections. Although the U.S. military bases are now closed, they have left this legacy behind. In

Olongapo and Angeles, where the bases were located, approximately 25,000 licensed hospitality women and thousands of other freelance workers served the rest-and-recreation needs of U.S. military personnel.

Female commercial sex workers, estimated to number between 200,000 and 500,000, are stigmatized by their work, class origins, rural backgrounds, and, lately, HIV. They have often been the objects of collective denial by both government and the public. Although the majority of sex workers are female, clandestine male brothels are found in all major urban centres. Many male sex workers also work out of gay bars and massage parlours offering "special services." An undetermined number of male sex workers solicit customers near commercial centres, cinemas, parks, and public toilets. A significant percentage of their clients are women.

Numbed by alcohol or drugs or lured by the money, many workers in the commercial sex industry easily succumb to unsafe sexual behaviour. Anything goes if the price is right, including sex without condoms. For many, the risk of infection is far less frightening than the immediate threat of hunger; becoming bedridden may take five to eight years, but their hungry stomachs must be filled today. The response of one female commercial sex worker is sadly typical of this pervasive fatalism: "I've been selling my body for five years. If HIV has been going around here, I'm sure I would have caught it. But I don't care."

Gays in the Philippines have also been stigmatized by their negative classification since the arrival of HIV. There is a large gay population in the Philippines and, despite the Catholic Church's official stance, homosexuality is not illegal. Activism has been slow to build because the gay community is disorganized and divided by the same class divisions, discrimination, and racism found in the heterosexual community.

The gay community's reaction to the crisis has ranged from disavowing any responsibility to accusing others. Some believe that sex workers and foreigners are to blame for the virus' spread. One prominent homosexual man even suggested that "low-class gays should be rounded up for testing, since they're the only ones who sleep with foreigners." The owner of a male brothel accepts long-term but not recent expatriates as clients, on the assumption that they are "clean." Even many "call boys" have begun to shun foreigners, who used to be their favoured clients.

All this is evidence of the social havoc caused by the disease among those labelled as high-risk in the Philippines. This categorization has resulted in further stigmatization of people already burdened by the moral prejudices of society. Yet little has been done to promote general awareness and to change sexual behaviour.

The growing scarcity of decent-paying jobs and the ever-growing labour force make it tempting for young men and women to capitalize on their bodies. A shadow population of hundreds, perhaps thousands, of children and adolescents who occasionally engage in the sex trade already exists. There are children who exchange sex for trips abroad or household appliances, as well as those who sell themselves for a meal or a pair of shoes. Many young people, especially boys from middle-class families, resort to occasional sex work when pressured by their peers to prove, ironically enough, their manhood or to provide money for the group.

The burgeoning group of sexually active children, adolescents, and young adults, many of whom have little knowledge about safe sex, makes the Philippines a nation ripe for catastrophe. Many will be exposed to HIV infection while fulfilling their sexual urges or struggling to survive. They are an elusive group that is not easily counted or identified, not easily contacted by educational campaigns. It will be even more difficult to reach young males who chauvinistically reject condoms. Few will consent to testing, and fewer still will acknowledge that they are infected, for fear of being ostracized by their peers.

Although commercial sex work is illegal, the government has devised intervention efforts targeting commercial sex workers as part of its national HIV/AIDS programme. Although the government is accelerating its drive to identify those affected by the disease, it has yet to implement a viable plan to care for the sick and the dying. In the interim, many who are already infected may be driven underground, becoming even harder to reach. Already there is resistance to testing among sex workers.

The Department of Health has created programmes to inform the public about the nature and transmission of HIV. Print and broadcast educational programmes have begun to confront some myths surrounding the disease. Telephone hot lines and television phone-in programmes have been helpful in answering questions.

The Catholic Church has planned its own intervention efforts and has mapped out an educational programme for schools and the population as a whole. Counselling, care, and alternative income sources for infected people are part of its provisions.

Nongovernmental organizations and other groups have sprouted up almost overnight to address the need for more immediate HIV and AIDS care. Artists have formed an organization called Reachout using theater, literature, and other art forms to inform the public about the issues. A number of private organizations are implementing intervention work among commercial sex workers. And gay men are finally banding together to form HIV support and informational groups, among them, the Library Foundation and the Gay Response to AIDS Prevention and Education (GRAPE).

The use of condoms must be an integral part of any HIV prevention programme. Yet here in the Philippines, resistance is high. Sometimes commercial sex workers, fearful that their clients will consider them diseased or dirty, shy away from using condoms. Filipino men are equally if not more resistant to their use for similar reasons and because they believe that condoms diminish pleasure.

Many Filipinos continue to regard condoms merely as contraceptives and not as barriers to sexually transmitted infections and HIV. The belief that ordinary hygienic measures such as washing the genitals before and after sex can prevent gonorrhea, syphilis, and HIV infection is still strong. Most people also assume that taking vitamins, having regular checkups, exercising, maintaining a proper diet, and, of course, praying are all effective HIV prevention methods.

Much of the resistance to condoms stems from their use as contraceptives and is centered in the Church. In a Catholic country struggling to deal with the problem of HIV, no issue is more controversial. The Catholic Church forbids artificial methods of birth control, despite galloping population statistics. The Vatican has condemned the use of condoms even for disease prevention. Consequently, the government, faced with the all-powerful Archbishop Jaime Cardinal Sin, has found it difficult to launch a full-scale safer-sex programme.

The pope maintains that HIV can be defeated only by a resurgence of moral values. But how can we stop commercial sex work? Unless we eliminate poverty, the basic reason for its existence, we will never have this "moral regeneration." Calling for a moral renewal instead of advocating practical means of combating the spread of HIV ignores the social, economic, and medical realities and the urgency of the crisis.

This is no time for ideological bickering. What the Filipino people need is a decisive and concerted effort to face the problem in all its varied ramifications. We do not need the veil of ideological vagaries and abstract mysticism. We must not wait until the epidemic begins to take a heavy toll on both our population and our economy.

Young, sexually active Filipinos are at risk. They are the country's labour force. We are also financially dependent on foreign investments and tourism, all of which would undoubtedly fall off if there were a large-scale epidemic. It is ironic that tourism is partially to blame for the problem but remains one of the country's major means of survival. Last, what are the ramifications for a government that is already cash-strapped? How will we be able to cope with the economic demands posed by a large-scale epidemic?

Now that the U.S. military bases have been dismantled, thousands of commercial sex workers, some of whom are already HIV-positive, are leaving Olongapo and Angeles to seek work in other urban and rural areas. It is becoming even more difficult to gain access to and empower them. The possibility of containing HIV infection within those areas will be lost. Inevitably, the disease will spread, cutting across gender and class lines and geographic regions.

If intervention programmes are to be successful, they must provide more than information and education. We must empower people to believe that they shape their own destinies, that what they do makes a difference, that HIV is not God-given. We found this approach effective in battling the political dictatorship. We can rekindle this spirit in our efforts to stop HIV.

We must tap into existing cultural values like the spirit of *tulungan*, which fosters concern for and participation in any community undertaking. Filipinos are, deep at heart, a communal people. They will lend a hand to someone in distress.

When and if the situation worsens, there is the spirit of *damayan*, oneness in the community. One demonstrates *damayan* by aiding the bereaved and aggrieved, by carrying the burden of one's fallen neighbour. The media have called on these traits many times in soliciting support for victims of natural calamities. We must draw on these values again in our fight against HIV.

Several miles outside of Manila, a volcano that had been dormant for more than 600 years erupted in 1991, claiming hundreds of lives and forcing thousands to flee. HIV, like Mount Pinatubo, will lie dormant, without signs or symptoms, for years. In those years of silence, the virus will build up its strength. One day it will erupt, not as spectacularly as Pinatubo, but far more fatally.

How much time is left before it will be too late to stop the disease from erupting? What will happen to people like Elmer and their families? What will happen to Filipino society? What measures are in place to forestall this major catastrophe? How prepared are the people? The alarm bell is ringing.

Although we have painted a grim scenario here, we still believe that all is not lost. We are not a hopeless lot. We are a nation of survivors who are resilient in the face of disaster. We can be shaken out of our apathy, as dramatized by the 1986 People's Power Revolution that toppled the Marcos regime. Ours was a revolution that served as a model for Eastern Europe's struggle for democracy. HIV demands that we organize a new revolution if we are to effectively control and prevent the spread of this disease. The future is in our hands.

5   The Economics of HIV Transmission

Deborah K. Raditapole

Deborah K. Raditapole is Minister of Health and Social Welfare in Lesotho. Previously, she was a pharmacologist and managing director of Materia Medica (Pty.) Ltd., a Lesotho-based company providing consultancy services in health and drug-supply management.

Migration and widespread population displacement in Lesotho are conditions that enable the spread of HIV and significantly increase women's risk of contracting the virus. Poor economies in the frontline states compel many young, able-bodied men to seek employment in South Africa. Migrant labour has become the mainstay of that country's mining industry and a critical component of its labour market.

Mobility—for example, the movement of people along major trade routes—plays a key role in the spread of HIV. The migrant labour system of South Africa involves the mobilization of hundreds of thousands of men from throughout the frontline states. In 1986, approximately 2.6 million workers were officially registered as migrants from areas within South Africa, excluding the independent homelands. An additional 378,000 foreign migrants were nationals of Lesotho, Mozambique, Malawi, Botswana, Swaziland, Zimbabwe, and Zambia.

Migrants throughout the world suffer stigmatization by their host country's population, but this sense of otherness is heightened by the political and social conditions that exist in

South Africa. They live apart from their families and traditional communities, in a racially polarized society, within confined living conditions. In this environment, feelings of isolation and loneliness increase, social constraints tend to diminish, and sex often becomes a source of escape and temporary solace.

In 1986, the South African government began random testing of miners for HIV. There was a high incidence of HIV among the Malawian mine workers, and the government repatriated all Malawians who tested positive. The government stated that it believed that the mass repatriation would slow down the spread of the disease. The miners, however, believed that the South African government was using HIV as an excuse to limit their numbers.

Forty per cent of South Africa's approximately 750,000 miners are foreign migrants, and the majority of them come from Lesotho. Among Lesotho's male working population, more than half the men are registered as migrant workers in South Africa, and many of them are married. The majority spend an average of fifteen years away from home, and nearly a third spend between seventeen and twenty-five years of their lives in the mines. Many leave home and never return. Some die in the mines, and some are killed amidst the violence that erupts in the camps; others simply start new families in neighbouring areas.

In Lesotho and throughout southern Africa, the migrant labour system encourages relationships that lead to the contraction and transmission of HIV. Miners live in poverty in crowded singles hostels removed from family, culture, and community. Long separations strain marriages, leaving both men and women open to extramarital relations. The sex industry in southern Africa is accessible in the border towns that miners travel through, where drinking, gambling, and sex serve as outlets to release tension or simply as activities to while away the time.

With so many men working outside the country, Lesotho now has a population made up of women, children, the elderly, and a few men who are often ill or incapacitated as a result of their prior employment in the mines. The government of Lesotho has become dependent on the easy and steady revenue received through the remittances of the migrant mine workers. Their absence also reduces the pressure on the government to address the issue of job creation at home. Lesotho's dependence on the income from migrant labour undermines its drive to develop alternative economic solutions.

Another outcome of the current labour system is that investment schemes in Lesotho that require significant numbers of workers must often import labour from neighbouring countries. These men, from as far north as Malawi and Zambia, also leave wives and families behind. Often these schemes are located in poor, mountainous areas of the country, where the lack of employment has encouraged young men to leave for long periods of time. These conditions have combined to institutionalize a geographic network of relationships that facilitate the spread of HIV.

Given the high prevalence of sexually transmitted infections, the numbers of migrant mine workers, and the simultaneous increase in HIV infection in neighbouring countries, it is likely that Lesotho will experience a dramatic rise in the occurrence of HIV as compared to what has been reported by the government to date. Effective education and prevention programmes are desperately needed for migrant workers. Their suspicions and doubts about the epidemic must be overcome. In addition to providing information and addressing individual behaviour, attention must be paid to the conditions that foster the behaviour that puts people at risk.

Many miners' wives are aware that their husbands' behaviour exposes them to HIV. These women voice concerns about men who use commercial sex workers and about the unsafe sexual practices that occur in the all-male singles hostels. Left to shoulder the responsibility of raising children and cultivating crops, these women are subject to oppressive cultural and traditional practices that leave them vulnerable to many forms of abuse. In Lesotho, a woman is still governed in most aspects of her life by customary law, under which she is regarded as a perpetual minor, subservient to her father's authority until she marries, and to her husband's authority thereafter. In his absence, control passes to the in-laws and remains with them if he dies. A husband has complete authority over his wife and may punish her as he sees fit. Wife beating is regarded as a disciplinary measure, not a crime.

Having sex with her husband is considered a wife's duty, even when she knows that her husband has had other partners and wishes to protect herself. If she insists that he use a condom or refuses to have sex with him, she may be beaten or abandoned. Even if a woman suspects that her spouse may have been exposed to HIV, she has nowhere to turn for support, and there are no laws to protect her.

In Lesotho, women's survival options are limited, even under the best of circumstances. A girl who gets pregnant while still in school is denied all chances of advancement. She is discriminated against by society and loses her self-esteem. Here, as in other countries, women benefit least from national social services. As a result, their poor education and scarce work opportunities allow few choices for survival. Widows in Lesotho usually turn to making and selling the local alcoholic brew to survive. Sex work, which is legal, becomes the only means of subsistence for many women. Some turn to sex work as a means of augmenting other income, because standard women's wages, which are usually lower than men's wages, are generally insufficient for their needs.

Our society condemns women for engaging in commer- cial sex work, but it ignores the economic, social, and cultural factors that encourage this activity. Many miners' wives are widowed at a young age and left with children to support. The culture does not give a widow the option of remarrying, thus sex work may be the only way a woman can earn enough to support her family. Lesotho's discriminatory laws restrict women's choices and access to income, thus limiting their options for survival.

Many women believe that miners should be given homes where they could live with their families. Although this would be an ideal situation, the process of its acceptance and implementation is dependent on the political system in South Africa. Poor Lesotho women have little, if any, direct influence on politics at home or in South Africa. They would rather cry out for the creation of jobs in Lesotho and thus decrease dependence on jobs in the mines.

Women are also likely to contract HIV from contaminated blood. They are exposed to the country's unsafe blood supply more often than men. This is especially true for malnourished, anaemic women who receive transfusions after childbirth. During delivery, women who are infected with HIV pose a risk to the traditional birth attendants who assist in 40 to 60 per cent of all home births. These attendants, mostly rural women whose hands and bodies are often scratched, cut, and scraped from manual labour, have limited, if any, access to rubber gloves.

Our society and our government must begin to address the impact of HIV on women for many reasons. A significant increase in HIV infection among women would deal a severe blow to both social and economic development in Lesotho.

In addition to providing food and shelter for their families, women's labour substantially contributes to the construction of roads, schools, and clinics. They also make up the majority of primary school teachers and workers in the health-care professions.

As caretakers of the family, women provide the first level of health care as well as moral and psychological support in times of illness. It is apparent that, as the HIV epidemic spreads, even greater demands are being placed on women. They now have the additional physical and psychological burden of attending to men who have become ill and return home to their villages to die. So far, little attention has been paid to the issue of caregivers for women and their dependents as they become ill.

With women functioning as the heads of households in a majority of homes, many children will become parentless as their mothers die of HIV-related illnesses. At present, these children are cared for by their extended families. As their numbers increase, it will become apparent that the government has made no provision for addressing the needs of these children. Significant outside investment of financial and human resources will be needed to cope with this aspect of the epidemic.

Despite the crucial role of women in Lesotho society, they are routinely stripped of their self-confidence. They have been so weakened by the system that they do not know how to organize themselves into effective pressure groups to fight for their rights. Now, more than ever, we must encourage women's self-confidence to enable them to bring about the changes that will meet their needs. This mobilization must begin in families, schools, churches, and communities. Young girls should be taught that they have a contribution to make to society and that they must take control of their lives.

HIV transmission cannot be controlled and reduced by information, education, and change of sexual behaviour alone. It is necessary to address the socioeconomic and political conditions that enable the spread of the epidemic. Rather than focus on and sometimes condemn individual behaviour, our strategy must place sexual behaviour in its social context. The economic culture spurred by the migrant labour system has removed much of our population from the safety of extended family and community support and replaced this with nothing.

Most of our education and prevention programmes are modeled on Western standards and are either poorly conceived or culturally unacceptable or inapplicable. If intervention programmes are to be successful, potentially dangerous cultural practices must be addressed in a manner that takes cultural norms into consideration. For example, in Lesotho, it is unacceptable for young women to speak about sexual issues with men, yet most of our nurses and health educators are young women. Special efforts must also be made to reach and involve our elders, because their word carries weight within the community.

We must move away from the language of crisis and catastrophe that has permeated the discussion of HIV. People will change their attitudes and behaviour not because of frightening information but because of positive messages that offer hope. We need to develop material that emphasizes hope rather than hopelessness.

Most of Lesotho's population is Christian, but we have not fully utilized the church's influence on our society. Many of us still see HIV as God's punishment for sins committed and show little sympathy for those infected. The church is in a strong position to take the lead in informing and educating society about HIV. It could help eliminate many of the myths surrounding HIV. Will HIV have to reach epidemic proportions before people own up to it?

Women are our greatest resource, and the church should come forward in support of women. It must champion women's cries for job creation and other social and economic changes that will encourage family stability. Who is there to listen to the cries of these women and wives? Often their voices go unheard within our communities.

It is critical that government review and address the conditions that discriminate against women. These conditions reduce women to mere commodities, diminish their self-esteem, and foster an environment that increases their risk of infection. This is an issue of human rights. Laws must be changed and introduced in support of these rights. The legal system, which still regards women as minors with little or no recourse to the law, must be restructured to minimize women's risk of contracting HIV. Efforts must be made to inform and educate women about laws that can help them, especially as they relate to marriage or abuse. Ethical and operational issues should be reexamined to take into account women's social and economic vulnerabilities. We must also work to control migrant workers' abandonment of families, even if the government does not believe that there is an urgent need to create more jobs at home or to change migration policy.

The intervention strategies of existing and future HIV control programmes need to recognize the unique situation of women and children. Empathy should be the key word. If women's concerns are not recognized and they are not incorporated into our HIV prevention programmes, we will lose our strongest allies and any hope for success as we face this challenge.

6   On the Eve of Destruction

Marie St. Cyr-Delpe

> Marie St. Cyr-Delpe is director of Iris House, an
> organization in New York servicing women infected with
> HIV. Previously, she was a deputy commissioner for
> community relations at the New York City Commission
> on Human Rights. She has been the director of the
> Haitian Coalition on AIDS, executive director of Women
> and AIDS Resource Network (WARN), and a consultant
> to the American Foundation for AIDS Research.

HIV, which knows no social or economic barriers, no
political ideology, and recognizes no skin colour, is planting
seeds of destruction in communities, nations, and continents
throughout the world. Yet each nation must face the challenge in the context of its own historical, cultural, economic,
social, and political realities.

The realities that shape the course of HIV in Haiti are devastating. The Haitian people have endured five decades of auto-
cratic rule, disastrous economic policies, environmental decay,
and social neglect. For much of this period, Haiti has been in
the midst of the most destructive political upheavals of its history. Just as the forests that once blanketed the hillsides have
been depleted, so too have the ranks of Haiti's citizens. Death
claims many as a result of endemic poverty, hunger, disease,
and political violence. Woefully inadequate health care has left
Haiti with one of the world's highest infant and maternal
mortality rates and an average life expectancy of fifty-five years
of age. Seventy-eight per cent of the population lives in poverty.

Given this situation, it is not surprising that Haitians have
fled the country in ever-increasing numbers. Beginning in

1957, with the advent of the Duvalier regime, Haiti began to experience a marked surge in emigration. It was the literate, educated, and skilled who began the exodus, but by the end of the Duvaliers' thirty-year reign, rural farmers, who had once migrated to the coastal cities, were leaving the country in growing numbers. Although many Haitians settled in other Caribbean nations or in Canada or Europe, the United States was the prime destination. As a result, there are more Haitian physicians in New York City than in Port-au-Prince.

The last ten years of the Duvalier regime and its aftermath—a period plagued by ever-changing civil-military governments—unfortunately coincided with the accelerated global spread of HIV. Throughout the 1980s, there was persistent denial of the dimensions of the HIV epidemic, first by government leaders and then by the people. Thus the changes needed to prevent the epidemic's spread were never addressed.

This denial was linked to the country's need to preserve its tourism industry, which was already suffering because of the deteriorating political climate. It was also fueled by the ruling elite's blatant disregard for the well-being of the majority of the Haitian people. But the level of denial among Haitians living at home and abroad was greatly increased by the stigmatizing link between Haiti and HIV globally, most notably in the United States. Therefore, HIV and AIDS were added to the list of taboos and family secrets, and the struggle for national dignity and personal pride overrode the need to develop prevention programmes.

Haiti is the only country once included by the United States' Centers for Disease Control in their "4H" categorization of groups at high risk of contracting and spreading the infection (homosexuals, heroin addicts, haemophiliacs, and Haitians). Thus, in 1982, Haitians who had immigrated to the

United States after 1977 were automatically barred from donating blood. By the time this classification was rescinded in 1990, Haitians had been irrevocably linked with HIV in the minds of many people. This stigma was also exacerbated by sensationalized stories in the global media that attempted to place the disease's origin in Haiti.

The Health Crisis and the Haitian Economy

The nation's denial of its HIV problem, along with the country's rapid economic, political, and social deterioration, all combined to set the stage for the current catastrophic health crisis. In mid-1991, Daniel Henrys, who was then Haiti's Minister of Health, acknowledged the need to integrate HIV into the country's health programme, but he said that HIV and AIDS fell last on the list of the nation's priorities, after malnutrition, tuberculosis, leprosy, diarrhoea, and infant and maternal mortality. He admitted that due to the government's lack of attention, the overall impact of HIV in Haiti would result in greater losses.

To better understand the potential impact of HIV on development in Haiti, consider the following. It has been estimated that 1 million Haitians now live abroad, and the numbers continue to grow. The majority of those departing are adults in the most productive stage of life—the age group most vulnerable to HIV. Those whom the society does not lose to emigration may be lost to HIV. Thus emigration and HIV are interwoven, as both are critical factors in the skilled-resource crisis that confronts Haiti today. Given the nation's low literacy rate and life expectancy, this crisis would worsen even if HIV were to be stopped in its tracks today.

As a result of the migration of rural people to coastal cities, lifestyles and sexual behaviour have changed. The majority of rural migrants were single. In the overcrowded, poor urban communities to which they moved, serial monogamy and sex with different partners—practices frowned upon in rural communities—frequently became a way of life. The intensifying economic hardship during the last decade has led to an increase in male and female commercial sex work.

Many studies have shown that a significant number of women are infected with HIV. This is of particular importance to the economy, because young, unmarried women constitute the overwhelming majority of employees who work on the assembly lines in Haiti's factories.

The private sector reinvests very little in Haiti, and most Haitian wealth is in foreign banks. The HIV epidemic is fostering a situation in which both the private and public sectors must share the responsibility of curbing the spread of this virus. The government's failure to respond to the epidemic has already compelled many employers to sponsor their own HIV and AIDS education programmes. These efforts are extremely important, but unfortunately, their agendas are often set by people who have neither the expertise in HIV prevention nor, in the case of many foreign employers, any actual knowledge of or abiding interest in the people.

It does not appear that current employer involvement is comprehensive enough to offset the spread of HIV. Workers are not passing the information on to their families. When employers begin to lose increasing numbers of their workers and experience a marked decline in productivity, they might consider coercive policies such as mandatory testing prior to hiring. Efforts must be made to ensure that such drastic policies are not implemented. At the same time, employers need to be provided with models for effective prevention programmes.

The Impact of Culture

Given that the majority of people who are infected with HIV may not know that they are seropositive or may not have changed their behaviour, Haiti's future is already being shaped by HIV. The social significance of the numbers of infected persons is profound. How many children will be left parentless and without care? How many families will be wiped out? How many thousands of people will be left destitute? What of the psychological impact on the survivors? Because Haiti's population is young, and because the disease affects those at the height of their reproductive and productive work years, the impact will be felt as support, purchasing power, and access to health care diminish.

This scenario, however, must not undermine our ability to search for alternatives that can defray the epidemic's impact on the future of our nation. Granted, we are starting this search late, but even if a vaccine were developed now, it would not necessarily eliminate HIV's presence in our midst. Therefore, we must develop strategies that will have a positive impact on the future.

Culture is at the core of our struggle against HIV in Haiti and the rest of the world, because our hopes for the future are anchored on changing attitudes and sexual behaviour. Personal, religious, and social beliefs must be taken into account. In Haiti, major change can occur only if prevention is integrated with traditional culture and values. The *hougans* (highest-ranking voodoo priests), the *bokos* (voodoo priests associated with spells and curses), Catholic priests, teachers, the press, and our political leaders must all be incorporated into this effort.

Urban and rural Haiti are as different as separate countries: their worldviews, cognitive processes, value judgments, and perceptions of government are not the same. Those involved in HIV education must create programmes that are designed specifically for each of these two different existences. In the rural areas, these programmes must be linked to the workplace, farm, and market square. They should also involve major institutions, places of worship, community leaders, and the neighbourhood *lakou* and *katie* (housing organized according to family hierarchy and religious rituals). For the urban areas, programmes should utilize advertising and promotion from other countries (Haitians are enamoured of imported goods), mass media, and prominent citizens or government representatives.

The need to reach rural people effectively is especially important, given that they represent the overwhelming majority of the population and are responsible for feeding the nation. As HIV travels from urban to rural areas, consideration should be given to a reverse-trend educational strategy in an effort to stave off the epidemic's spread.

In order to devise effective prevention programmes, one must address socially sanctioned gender-based attitudes and behaviour. In Haiti, women are perceived as the vector of the disease. This perception is not limited to women who are commercial sex workers but applies to all sexually active women. Those who are known to be infected with HIV or AIDS are hardest hit by ostracism, hatred, and victimization. Along with women's low status in society and their culturally mandated social and sexual passivity, this stigmatization makes it virtually impossible for most Haitian women to initiate safer sex practices for fear of public censure and male reprisal. For many single women, sex with multiple partners and serial monogamous relationships have become necessary strategies for economic survival. This also leaves them particularly vulnerable to HIV infection. Regardless of marital status, a woman's ability to protect herself is inevitably linked to poverty and a culturally prescribed subservient role in society.

Despite the fact that economic realities and culturally sanctioned attitudes combine to prevent the empowerment of Haitian women when negotiating the terms of sexual conduct, HIV prevention is being focused on them. By failing to make the education of Haitian males the priority, prevention policies essentially absolve men of responsibility while reinforcing the belief that HIV is a woman's disease. Placing the burden of responsibility on women for preventing transmission is almost guaranteed to fail.

Prevention efforts in their current form are merely catering to prevailing beliefs. Educators' failure to rid themselves of these notions and their limited expertise present some of the gravest problems in HIV prevention. The unwillingness of officials to address the disease in a positive way exacerbates the situation. By continuing to downplay or deny the seriousness of the epidemic, they fail to provide the people with leadership in promoting behaviour change. If prevention is to succeed, educators should demonstrate greater awareness and devise relevant programmes that address traditional beliefs and values. They must focus their efforts on reaching men.

The other aspect of Haitian culture that influences education, prevention, and care is the interweaving of religious and ritual values with concepts of health and illness. Integral to the concept of illness and healing is the notion of the supernatural and of recourse to folk medicine for treatment. Surviving an illness is a collective activity among Haitians. When a person is ill, family and community are in continuous attendance, providing care, preparing strong food, and appealing to religion for healing. Fear of HIV is now eroding this psychological and physical support system. In its absence, patients tend to die sooner and alone. Their children are avoided, and instead of the acclamation that traditionally follows a death, there is only silence.

Change Is Inevitable

Because HIV challenges the accepted notion of healing, in Haiti the epidemic undermines the deification of doctors as well as the traditional healers. Long-held traditions and the underlying economic exploitation by healers will be questioned. Traditional approaches to healing may be merged with Western medicine to enhance people's knowledge, diminish the competition between the two methods, and provide validation for both. It is hoped that there will be family involvement in the medical care of patients with HIV-related illnesses, because the country's health-care institutions are ill equipped to manage the increasing numbers of these patients.

Inevitably, HIV creates fear that affects sexuality. The administration of President Aristide, which reflects the morality of the Catholic Church and preaches the need to respect and protect families, may provide leadership in advocating behaviour change. Although I do not believe that Haitians will ever return to the staid sexual patterns of the past, more responsible sexual behaviour can occur. To achieve this, the government and private sector must make special efforts.

Students and educators should be trained and must spend time in the provinces sharing information with youngsters.

Haitians living abroad with skills in counselling or medicine should be recruited as volunteers to train others and to work in the field. Specific programmes geared to the education of the unemployed and those living in poverty should also be priorities. Neighbourhood teach-ins should utilize and include people from within the community as educators.

I am often reminded of a statement made by Zambia's former president, Kenneth Kaunda: "The most important thing is not to know where the disease comes from but to discover where it is going." We must acknowledge and confront the reality of our situation. By honestly evaluating what the outcome may be, we can move decisively to reduce the negative impact, using strategies based on traditions and values that shape our lives.

HIV mirrors the inequities of the world. Inevitably, the epidemic's true impact on developing nations can be offset only if the crisis compels world leaders to respond with compassionate programmes that hold life more dear than the strategic economic and political manifestations of power. A comprehensive global approach, one that fully marshals the world's material and intellectual resources to fight HIV, is the only method through which we all truly stand a chance of reducing the destructive impact of the epidemic.

7   Our Future Is at Stake

Robert E. S. Mugemana

*Robert E. S. Mugemana instituted the HIV programme
of the Norwegian Church Aid Society in Nairobi, Kenya,
and later worked as a consultant for the UNDP HIV
and Development Programme. He was a freelance
journalist who received his training at the University College of Eastern Africa in Kenya and the
Africa Literature Centre in Zambia. Mugemana
married in 1991. He died of AIDS in 1993.*

When I began writing this article, I decided to return to a
brothel I had patronized during my last year of secondary school,
fully expecting that with the advent of HIV it would be closed.
I was in for a shock, because not only was it fully operational,
but business was booming. The older women were gone,
replaced by girls as young as fourteen and no older than twenty-
five. I had to push my way through a crowd of men in the
corridor. Most of the customers were young men in their twenties and early thirties; there were schoolboys, university students,
civil servants, and others, from all walks of life.

One of the girls and I went to the bar to talk. After
exchanging a few pleasantries, I asked if she had any condoms.
She replied that she did, but I would have to pay extra for
them. If I did not wish to pay for the condom, we could have
sex without using one. I asked her if she was afraid of contracting HIV. "Well," she said, then thought for a minute and
replied uncomfortably, "You cannot do this kind of business
if you fear that disease."

As we continued our conversation, I inquired about the
number of clients she had sex with on an average day. She

told me, "The week before and after the end of the month, when business is good, I can have fifteen in one night." When I asked if any of them used condoms, she said, "Two or three, and usually they are married. They fear contracting gonorrhea from us and passing it on to their wives."

I spoke with four more of her colleagues, who all seemed to think that it was the man's responsibility to protect himself. They did not protect themselves from their clients because they all shared a sense of fatalism about becoming infected. As one of them said, "Even if HIV was not there, I would die anyway." A similar attitude is evident among many young people. When they discover that former lovers have died from HIV-related diseases, they fear that they could be infected but prefer not to be tested and know for sure. Instead, they keep their fears to themselves.

There are many brothels in Nairobi that are providing much-needed income for many women. Girls who have dropped out of school due to pregnancy or because they lack the resources to continue their education often turn to sex work as a means of survival. And for men who leave their wives behind in the rural areas while they pursue employment in the cities, brothels offer an inexpensive source of sexual activity. In fact, this activity is now one of the major modes of HIV transmission. At the end of each month, men return to their villages with the money they have earned in the urban areas. They may be infected with HIV, and many unknowingly infect their wives.

Visiting brothels or having girlfriends while married is fairly common for Kenyan men. With the advent of HIV, their behaviour places them, their families, the other women they come in contact with, and the entire society at risk. When a forty-nine-year-old friend of mine recently died of HIV-related illnesses, he left behind two wives—one in the village with six children, and the other in Nairobi with four children. All ten children were in school. He was also responsible for his elderly parents and occasionally contributed school fees for a few of his in-laws' children. The entire extended family depended on him. He died without informing either of his wives that he had contracted HIV, and now his wife in Nairobi has developed herpes zoster and oral thrush.

My late friend held a senior position in a large company, and during his burial, the managing director was visibly shaken by my friend's untimely death. In the same company, out of a total workforce of 185 people, at least fourteen others have contracted HIV, including three senior and five middle managers. Each of these employees, regardless of rank, is an important asset to the company. These fourteen decided to be tested after experiencing symptoms of HIV-related illnesses, but who knows how many other employees, knowingly or unknowingly, are living with HIV.

Now that my friend is gone, who will provide for his children? He left enough money to cover the next two years' school fees, but once those resources are exhausted, who will step in and provide for the extended family? Where will his wife in Nairobi find money for treatment now that she is ill? How long will it take the company to replace him? How much future productivity has the company lost in terms of the substantial investment it made in him? Should the company begin training new personnel to take over the jobs of HIV-positive employees who can no longer carry out their duties satisfactorily? Should all prospective employees be tested for HIV prior to hiring? And what of the other families and companies in similar and far worse situations?

This is not an isolated case. In my career as a counsellor, I have worked with hundreds of clients, and it frightens me to see how HIV is stealing the most productive men and women in our society. I have seen doctors, lawyers, engineers, farmers, pilots, educators, legislators, clergymen, and people from all walks of life succumb. They are leaving behind a large gap that will surely be impossible to fill in the near future. Undoubtedly this will adversely affect development. The magnitude of the situation is yet to be felt, but as more people contract HIV, we will certainly experience a critical shortage of skilled labour.

It is also important to remember that agriculture forms the backbone of Kenya's economy. The group most affected, those aged eighteen to forty-five, is the same group that farms the land and feeds the nation. If the present rate of infection is not halted, Kenya, which has been nearly self-sufficient agriculturally, will soon have to import food.

Will Kenya survive the onslaught of HIV? Five years ago, I would have thought that question preposterous and dismissed it. Now, virtually every Kenyan has heard of HIV, how one becomes infected, and what to do to prevent transmission. This awareness, however, has had little impact on the spread of HIV thus far. What worries me most is that more than 90 per cent of those infected with the virus do not know that they are infected.

Our nation has the capacity and the infrastructure to contain this epidemic. However, the breakdown of our social structure has reached almost irreversible proportions. This has been exacerbated by authoritarianism, the greatest threat to social justice and empowerment. People must have complete freedom to make positive and informed decisions about their lives. This is the only way that they will be able to take preventive action against HIV. Unfortunately, this is not the case for Kenyans at this time.

But all may not be lost if the government puts HIV at the top of its agenda. Key ministries must take the lead by setting aside at least 10 per cent of their budgets for HIV prevention programmes in their areas of operation. For example, the Ministry of Education should ensure that teachers and students, from the elementary level to the university level, are reached throughout the country. Meanwhile, international aid donors should move to strengthen their commitments—financial and otherwise—to local nongovernmental organizations involved in HIV prevention. These organizations not only seem to be doing more than the government itself, but they are also more accountable and efficient.

We should stop emphasizing the word *AIDS* and instead focus on the term *HIV*. When we tell people that anyone could be carrying HIV, we must provide them with counselling and information to counteract their belief that only those who are thin and emaciated can transmit the virus. It is the person with HIV who is healthy, sexually active, and unaware that he or she is transmitting the virus to others, as well as those who are uninfected, whom we should be concerned about.

To reach them, we must use prevention programmes that are specific to Africa rather than instituting programmes that have been created for Western countries and are inapplicable in Africa. The present programme in Kenya is disease-centred, and it should be refocused to become person-centred. The disease must be visualized to be understood fully. We must give HIV a human face in order to assist people in overcoming their fears. And we must ensure that each person who tests positive for HIV is provided with counselling services as a right, not as an obligation.

We have to admit and address a number of other HIV-enabling conditions, issues, and practices that provide fertile ground for the virus in our society. We cannot ignore the fact that older men are becoming sexually active with young girls as a means of preventing contraction of HIV, thus placing another generation at risk. We need to address traditional cultural practices, such as the circumcision of groups of boys and girls with one unsterilized blade. We must also examine the risks involved in ritual cleansing, where the closest male kin of a deceased husband has sex with the widow, and where one razor blade is used to make ritual incisions on the bodies of remaining family members. We must also confront and find ways to overcome people's reluctance to use condoms, along with their fatalism and refusal to accept the epidemic as a reality.

Needless to say, Kenyan society must change its views regarding the status of women. A woman—particularly in the rural areas, where the majority of our population lives—has no rights or direct income from her labour. She is like a slave, and this condition offers her little protection from HIV. As long as women remain in passive and subservient positions, they cannot question their husbands' sexual practices. Even when a wife is aware of her husband's involvement with another woman, she suffers in silence. Countless women who have never had sexual relations with men other than their husbands have become infected as a result of his behaviour.

When a husband becomes ill, it is the woman who nurses him. When a child is ill, it is the woman who nurses it. But when a woman is ill, she nurses herself. When a couple are both HIV-positive, often the husband dies before the wife. Thus the wife is left to struggle with their children, to endure and face stigmatization and isolation, and ultimately to face her own death alone. These women desperately need support and counselling. Something must be done to counter the prevailing belief that any incurable disease is a curse and the person affected should be left alone to die.

The majority of Kenyans are Christians. Our churches are extremely powerful, and they are much more vocal than government regarding the social issues of today. Yet this enormous power has not been used to educate their worshippers about the risks and dangers of HIV infection. We need the churches to use their privileged position and influence to prevail upon congregations to advocate prevention, put it into practice, and positively respond to those who are ill.

Kenyan society is fragmented due to a policy of divide and rule practiced by the colonialists for decades. Yet despite that fragmentation, families still retain a strong sense of identity and togetherness. In Kenya, one does not live as an individual but as part of a family. In times of need, one turns to one's family for support and care. African families traditionally care for their loved ones at home, especially the terminally ill. We must strengthen the family's capacity for caregiving as we begin to depend on them to care for those living with HIV. In two years, our hospitals and health-care institutions— already stretched to their limits—will be unable to accommodate the increasing number of patients with HIV-related illnesses. Home-based care is the only feasible solution. To cope with HIV, basic nursing skills should be incorporated into adult literacy classes, which are being conducted at the community level throughout the country.

Despite all the difficulties and pain this epidemic causes, there are some positive aspects to HIV. As people and communities recover from the initial shock of HIV and its effects, they have begun to band together and seek methods of caring for those of us living with HIV and AIDS. Also, single young men and women are getting married with the intention of committing to monogamous unions as a means of avoiding contracting HIV. Slowly, global connections are being made to meet the challenge of this epidemic. Perhaps most important, the epidemic has shown us that the world is indeed one family, equally vulnerable, and that human love knows no boundaries of nationality.

8 A Challenge to the Powerless Woman

Joan Ross-Frankson

> *Joan Ross-Frankson is a Jamaican journalist with some twenty years' experience in the fields of broadcasting, audio-visuals, print, research and documentation, and public relations. For the past nine years, she has worked almost exclusively within the Caribbean nongovernmental sector, assisting with the development of communications programmes and special publications.*

Five hundred years after Christopher Columbus bucked up on his way east, inflicting influenza and slave labour on the native Arawak Indians, global powers are still sneezing and the rest of us are still catching their colds. The advent of HIV and AIDS in the Caribbean is a new-age symptom of our historical position of powerlessness in a world where the hand of the rich controls the blade that slashes the hand of the poor. To tackle this problem on a local level, we of the developing countries must challenge this global status quo more aggressively than we are now doing. This is a time, and a disease, that feeds on the world's weak and vulnerable.

HIV was initially portrayed as a man's disease, an illness that affected only male homosexuals. Indeed, it was even promoted as a disease of American gays and drug users. Women, therefore, were lulled into a false sense of security. It is only recently that more accurate information is being disseminated about HIV transmission and how women are being affected.

Available data, including surveys among both high- and low-risk groups, suggest a 0.1 per cent infection rate, making it likely that some 2,500 Jamaicans have already been infected by HIV—and many do not even know it. Obviously, future news is not expected to be good. Even the most optimistic experts are projecting that within the next ten to fifteen years, AIDS will be killing an estimated 1,000 Jamaicans a year. And women are fast becoming the most HIV-endangered population group. Currently the male-female AIDS ratio in Jamaica is 2.5:1, a little less than the Caribbean average of 2:1. Into the new century, Jamaican women are expected to be on an equal 1:1 footing with their men. (*AIDS Window*, vol. 1, no. 1, Sept. 1990.) Jamaicans must be shocked into changing their sexual lifestyles today, before they become deathstyles.

For Jamaican women, whose economic powerlessness and lower social status often force them to accept rape in all its forms, the reality of HIV threatens to be severe. Burdens of domestic life will increase significantly as traditional responsibilities stretch to include taking care of those in our own families who are ill as well as the parentless children left behind by our sisters.

Twenty-seven-year-old Lil is from a low-income family in Jamaica's capital city, Kingston. She is woefully underemployed, doing a domestic day's work when she can get it. She relies on support from her aunt and her father to support herself and her six-year-old son. All four of them live in two apartments that are part of a tenement yard complex of old board shacks. Lil's brother came to live with the family when he became too weak from HIV-related illnesses to care for himself.

"It was a lot of extra physical work," Lil explained. "He wouldn't keep his area clean or go to the bathroom, and we were very crowded, so life was miserable. Trying to keep the place clean and get rid of the flies really got to me. Then there was so little money."

Junie is twenty-eight years old and unemployed. She comes from a large, close-knit family; she has one child of her own and is also caring for her sister's two daughters, who are both under five years old. Her sister died last year from an HIV-related illness. Junie and the family did not know that she had contracted HIV.

Junie describes her frustration at her sister's secrecy. "She died and she neva tell nobody, not even her madda. We feel bad about that. If she did tell us we would keep it secret, but she neva tell us. Her baby-father did migrate when the little one born and we can't hear nothing from him. But because I love her children I don't mind looking after them, and all the family help from the start until now."

As the number of HIV-positive women increases, many more will suffer the pain of birthing infected babies who die before their eyes. Many of us will wish our children dead even as we curse, in frustration and anger, the perceived source of our vulnerable and infected bodies.

Florris' anger is directed at her baby's father. Her son, Derron, seemed healthy at birth, but trouble signs began to appear before he was two months old. It was only after tests showed that he was HIV-positive that Florris found out that she was carrying the virus. "I was so angry, I wanted to kill the father," she said with deep feeling. Derron's father, Florris' only sexual partner at the time, refuses to believe that he passed the virus on to her and has continued his pattern of sexual conquest in business-as-usual style. "He wouldn't even get tested, can you believe that? There should be a law to force HIV-infected people to behave in a more responsible way," Florris said in anger.

Lana is thirty-six but looks more like fifty. She is barely literate, unemployed, and painfully thin. She tested positive for HIV when her fourth child was born with HIV. "He was seven month old when him dead and I said, 'Thank God!' when them tell me. It was hard, but I was looking forward to it because he was suffering so badly," she said with pain.

Until two years ago, Lascelles was working as an orderly at a public hospital and living with his male partner. Within six months, everything changed dramatically. His partner succumbed to HIV-related complications and Lascelles tested positive for HIV. "I was tested at the hospital where I worked, so in two-twos all the staff got to know about it," he explained. "I lost my job. People refused to work with me. Soon after, my partner died from AIDS, and the landlord threw me out. News travels fast in Jamaica."

Lascelles is now homeless and has been completely rejected by society. Forecasts point to a dramatic increase in the number of people living with HIV who will be left to wander the streets in the face of fear and prejudice from family, friends, employers, and landlords.

Public Education

These stories of anonymous individuals who have tested positive for HIV are poignant and run the gamut from bravery to bitterness, from fortitude to helplessness. Individual experiences with HIV are being used in the island's newspapers as a dramatic way of getting information about the disease to the population. But because Jamaican society is painfully class-biased and harbours deep racial contradictions and homophobic tendencies, only the lives of the most powerless are highlighted: low-income women and their children, working-class homosexuals, commercial sex workers, migrant farm workers, and petty traders.

If society's middle and upper classes, the educated, the policy makers, or the successful entrepreneurs have been touched by HIV, they are certainly not letting this information escape their closed circle. They get tested by private doctors and fly overseas for treatment, thus keeping their reputations intact and away from the fast-moving local *suss* (gossip) machine. They worry behind closed doors while society comforts itself that only the poor can become infected with HIV.

The Jamaican public has been warned that HIV kills and informed of the need to practice safe sexual habits. However, at this moment, HIV has been relegated to the pile of problems that will be tackled tomorrow. Just 250 deaths in nine years does not begin to measure up in the national consciousness with 207 violent killings in the first 122 days of 1991 or almost two road deaths a day in 1990 in a population of 2.5 million. And this is against a background of underdevelopment that is an awesome burden on us.

A Basket to Carry Water

Today's debilitating reality is our economic submission to the whip of massive external indebtedness. Structural adjustment policies imposed by the International Monetary Fund and the World Bank since 1979 have continually devalued the Jamaican dollar, imposed wage freezes, liberalized imports, removed government subsidies on basic food items, and cut back social services. The repayment of the debt requires more than half of all foreign exchange earned by the country and has drained the social services and the lives of all income groups except the most wealthy in our society.

Cutbacks in health services have already placed enormous constraints on our ability as a nation to face the advent of HIV and AIDS. These cutbacks affect workers in the public health system, who say that their task is like trying to carry water in a basket. The dismal picture in our hospitals and clinics is of low-level maintenance, lack of life-saving equipment, high-priced drugs, and inoperative surgical facilities.

These unhealthy conditions have been compounded by an exodus of nurses from the health-care system. Wage restraints have destroyed our nurses' ability to keep up with the leaping cost of living. The result is a health-care system that needs approximately 3,000 nurses to function efficiently but now depends on less than 1,000.

Rose, an intensive-care nurse, was on duty at the island's only teaching hospital when she decided to migrate. That day, the unit was full, and during Rose's shift a young woman, a boy, and an elderly man could not receive treatment and subsequently died. "I trained as a nurse to help save lives," she explained. "These conditions make it impossible for me to function professionally, and it is heartbreaking to watch so many die unnecessarily. Then on top of the heartache, I can't ever hope to own a house or a car. It is demoralizing."

Education has followed the same demoralizing pattern, with government spending consistently decreasing over the last decade. Worsening conditions and low salaries have robbed our classrooms of the best teachers as they resign at alarming rates. Thus teaching standards have fallen drastically, followed, inevitably, by poor student performance.

Neglect of small farming in favour of large-scale projects exporting solely to the U.S. market has brought about a sharp decline in the nutritional standards of our population. This has resulted in moderate to severe malnutrition in children under the age of five, as well as outbreaks of diseases such as measles, malaria, and typhoid, which were thought to have been eradicated during the 1970s.

Women Under Pressure

Jamaican women are at the centre of the country's economic storm. Exploitation of their time and labour is central to maintaining structural adjustment policies. Over half of our households are headed by women, and the remaining half rely heavily on women's incomes. In addition to propping up the collapsing health-care system, Jamaican women are trying to meet almost daily price increases while earning the lowest wages. Many are not able to meet these demands.

Cutbacks in health, education, and the garment industry—areas where women work in large numbers—have pushed many women out of work. Export-oriented production promoted by the International Monetary Fund and the World Bank has not absorbed them.

Myth and Sexuality

For women, economic powerlessness often goes hand in hand with sexual powerlessness. Most women are not independent enough to make sexual choices for their own benefit.

Jamaicans are sensual people. Men and women meet and exchange sexual sparks in every situation at all levels of society. The mutual consent of an eligible couple is all that is required to obtain social sanction for sexual relations. Sex is celebrated in song and dance, yet we are amazingly unsystematic when it comes to transmitting sexual knowledge.

Our only formally institutionalized mechanism for sex education is at the secondary school level under the misnomer of guidance counselling. With rare exceptions, parents do not discuss sexuality with their children, so it is not surprising that accurate knowledge of human anatomy is lacking in our society. Many believe that an intrauterine device or a condom can get lost in the body, that injection of the contraceptive drug Depo-Provera blocks the tubes and decreases fertility, and that a buildup of birth-control pills over time requires a good laxative to wash out the system. Although Jamaicans believe that sex is natural and healthy, they will also tell you that repression of this natural urge can cause headaches and mental stress and that too much sex can run down and harm the body.

During our socialization process, Jamaican females are at a distinct disadvantage. In the first few years of life, there is no sex-role differentiation, but by puberty, the activities of girls are sharply curtailed as parents make a conscious effort to teach them proper behaviour and modesty. Boys are encouraged to interact with others outside the home, but girls are severely restricted, watched, and controlled. Nonetheless, sex itself begins at an early age for both boys and girls. On average, a boy's age of first sexual encounter occurs when he is between fourteen and fifteen years of age; for a girl it occurs between age sixteen and seventeen. In the case of girls, attainment of a higher education is an important factor in delaying sexual activeness.

Safer Sexual Behaviour

Known locally as boots, condoms do not have many male friends in Jamaica. Although an increase in condom use has been observed recently, most Jamaicans believe that HIV is preventable without modifying sexual behaviour.

National HIV education programmes directed at the entire population have so far had little effect on beliefs regarding the disease. Programmes targeted toward commercial sex workers also ran into difficulties. The major problem was that the programmes were both sexist and classist in their approaches. They were sexist because they targeted female sex workers and ignored the men who paid for sex. They were classist because they targeted only street walkers, refusing to recognize the blurring of lines between women who are commercial sex workers and middle- and upper-class women who are more informal in their use of sex for economic gain.

Andrine, a thirty-four-year old sex worker explained how she entered the trade: "I've been a prostitute from ten years. I started cause me did need di money and me did have friends in the business who encourage me. The fathers of my two children did not help me and I wanted money to make sure they did not come like me. I leave school when I was thirteen, but right now I'm trying to do some English and some maths so I can manage better.

"I did try domestic work, but di little bit a money could never finance me like how I did want. It [prostitution] was nice at first, but den me start worry bout di danger you have to face from police and di customer dem. But worse was when me hear 'bout AIDS. Dat was in 1982. I hear bout it on di radio and read it in di *Gleaner*. Me did think first time dat it was only Americans who have it, and me did start use condom wid dem. But after looking deeper me realize di Americans come as tourists and they use prostitute and the prostitutes still have local customers, an' I get frightened.

"Me start use condoms with all a dem, local and foreign same way. But it's hard because some a di man dem have an attitude. Dem wan go bed with you but they doesn't want to use condom. Some of dem offer you extra money if you don't use the condom. Some a dem sneak and push hole inna di condom so it will burst out on you. Some of them, when dem dun, dem hold you down and tek back di money. Dem seh it nuh feel right wid condom and dem neva get dem money-worth.

"Most a we know we tek a risk without a condom, but if di man offer more money and tings working bad fi di night, well, you tek di extra money. Den you hafta spend it back on di doctor when you get sick.

"Me personally nuh tink it worth it. I would never want AIDS cause people would scorn me, and how would I cope with my children? Up to now, dem nuh know me a prostitute."

Andrine has made some choices to engage in safe sex or no sex at all. For a married woman or mistress, these choices may not exist. They are often unable to defend themselves when weakened by the sanctity of marriage and the privacy of the home.

One middle-class, married professional woman explained her inability to protect herself from HIV: "I know my husband is sleeping around, he always has. I thought when we were first married that he would change. Now I am at my wit's end with this AIDS business. I got so frightened I bought some condoms, but he refused to use them. He said I had no right to shortchange him on sex, and that there were plenty of women out there who would give him sex without condoms.

"I didn't challenge him because I don't want to lose him. How would I manage with the children on my salary? I'm sure he wouldn't help financially if we separated. So now we end up having sex, but I'm so afraid."

Sexual contact between men and women in any society is an outcome of a historical social, political, and cultural reality.

It is not that we Jamaican women have struggled any less to develop and protect the rights we have won for ourselves and our children. We too were "equal under the whip" during slavery, so I am optimistic that we will use our talents. I do not take a pessimistic view of this region's future vis-à-vis HIV. I am optimistic that women will use their talents to create positive changes for ourselves and our families.

Generally speaking, we Caribbean women have always been good at organizing ourselves. Our informal trading habits— going back to the days when we framed plots of land and travelled from the country to town, and across the waters, to sell our goods—are an essential part of Caribbean life. In parliamentary politics, we have been central to the process of change. We have served our political parties in many roles, though we have achieved little actual political power for our efforts. In church, we maintain the day-to-day operations, yet few women are present in the decision-making structure, and ordination of women to the priesthood is far from the normal practice.

At the social level, we are organized into groups that seek realistically priced housing, raise consciousness, expose and combat negative media images of women, and argue for our rights on all fronts. In recent years, lobbying efforts have expanded to the national level through an umbrella organization that seeks to change attitudes and practices relating to sexual violence, sex bias in the workplace, the cost of living, and many more issues of concern to women and men.

However, we have not made significant strides in relation to our bodies and our sexuality. This is why HIV is not yet a major issue within our women's movement. Will we wait until the disease affects us in larger numbers before we stop hiding behind the veil of secrecy, prejudice, and embarrassment? I think it is far more likely that we'll take action around

HIV and AIDS in a holistic way. This action is likely to include a stepped-up lobby for more meaningful sex education in our schools, for health workshops in which more of us can learn the facts about our bodies. But these and other actions can be successful only if we are involved in the overall political and economic decision-making machinery.

Dependency is a terrible thing for people and nations. Development is not just about land, capital, technology, and markets. It is also about the physical, psychological, and intellectual well-being of the labour force. Women's roles are essential precisely because they have the most to contribute to, and gain from, development that is based on people's needs. The social, economic, and political systems now in place work for only small sections of humanity. Because they are based on unequal power relations—whether between women and men, country and country, or people and nature—they simply cannot work for the vast majority. The HIV epidemic expresses the urgent need for humanity to address these imbalances.

9 Clients and Commercial Sex Work

Eka Esu-Williams

Dr. Eka Esu-Williams is a senior lecturer in the Department of Immunology at the University of Calabar. She is a founding member and the current president of the Society for Women and AIDS in Africa (SWAA) and is the AIDS programme coordinator for the Cross River State of Nigeria. She has extensive experience with HIV prevention programmes aimed at female commercial sex workers and their clients.

An accurate assessment of the scope and intensity of the HIV epidemic in Nigeria continues to be elusive, retarding the evolution of rational decisions and appropriate actions by health policy makers and other interested parties. The low numbers of cases reported to date reinforce the officially sanctioned notion of Nigeria as a country in which there is a low prevalence of HIV. This, in turn, reinforces the already pervasive apathy among the population, who believe that there is no significant present or future threat.

Recent surveillance studies offer a potentially more accurate picture of Nigeria's precarious position, documenting seroprevalence rates of up to 36 per cent among women working in the commercial sex industry, up to 5.8 per cent among prenatal clinic clients, and up to 4 per cent among blood donors. Among commercial sex workers in the city of Lagos, a baseline HIV prevalence of 3 per cent in 1987 rose to 17 per cent in 1992; among blood donors in Maiduguri City, it rose from 0 per cent in 1987 to over 4 per cent in 1992. Although this difference may be attributable to more intensive and regular testing, it is likely that new infections account for most of the dramatic increase.

These figures represent an exponential increase in infection rates. They suggest that HIV infection is entrenched in the population and is assuming epidemic proportions. Unfortunately, current attitudes and competing demands for scarce resources leave the Nigerian population vulnerable to a rapid spread of HIV infection and subsequently to AIDS.

The Cross River State (CRS) of Nigeria is one of the country's twenty-one states; it has a population of about 2 million out of a total 106 million nationwide. The CRS provides a prototype for targeted interventions. An HIV prevention programme for commercial sex workers and their clients started in 1987. The formulation and execution of the programme activities involved key members of the target group, such as hotel owners and managers, chairladies (head sex workers), sex workers, and clients. To indicate the programme's scope to date, a total of more than 1,500 low-income, full-time resident sex workers and clients have been reached.

Commercial sex work is not culturally sanctioned in Nigeria, and it is seldom a preferred choice of vocation. Women are commonly coerced into it for a variety of reasons, including involuntary divorce, widowhood, joblessness, and, in some cases, infertility. The CRS programme found no women for whom sex work was a choice rather than a necessity, and 95 per cent of them were prepared to abandon this occupation if alternative employment with comparable or even slightly lower income could be found.

Because sex work is illegal and highly stigmatized, female sex workers in Nigeria become part of a vicious circle of exploitation and harassment by their clients, hotel owners and managers, and law-enforcement agents. The latter have traditionally viewed them as easy targets for extortion. According to the women, one of the many unwritten rules is that the client is always right. This is rigidly enforced by hotel owners and managers to encourage a steady flow of clients, which in turn ensures that sex workers pay their bills. The clients often determine the price, and many claim dissatisfaction and seek a refund or later request compensation for treatment of a sexually transmitted infection (STI) without offering proof of infection. There is seldom an opportunity for the women to save money. In fact, the price for their services has remained the same for over a decade, despite spiralling inflation. Given these conditions, the women are compelled to seek and accept a high number of clients.

The inability to negotiate fairly with clients, hotel owners and managers, and law-enforcement agents, coupled with social stigmatization, leads to and perpetuates low self-esteem and group-esteem among the women. They commonly refer to one another as *ashawo,* a derogatory local name for a commerical sex worker, and to their children as *ashawo pikin.* They are reluctant to deal with decisions and transitions that affect their lives, particularly those involving persons in positions of authority.

The new, younger sex workers do not, however, abandon their desire for children. With little access to family planning and health information, these young women are at considerable risk of contracting HIV. They are also at risk of becoming pregnant, leading inevitably to an upsurge in the number of infants with HIV infection and paediatric AIDS cases.

Exploitation, extortion, negative self-perception, and societal condemnation ultimately disable many women working in the commercial sex industry. Often these attitudes render them incapable of reintegrating into society should they choose to disengage from the business. Those that remain are not equipped to seek and adopt the health-promoting behaviours necessary for HIV prevention.

In an effort to redress some of these inequities, the CRS programme staff involved law-enforcement agents, hotel owners and managers, and chairladies in an agreement to keep rents at current levels while allowing the women to charge more money for sex. As a result of this collaboration, harassment and extortion by law-enforcement agents have become rare, and we have seen new expressions of self- and group-confidence among the women, including more assertive negotiation for condom use.

Targeting Clients

Although commercial sex workers are readily identifiable, their clients often try to conceal their identities. The CRS programme gathered information about clients from managers, the sex workers themselves, and clients who volunteered. The men were primarily Nigerians and represented a cross section of the population, ranging from low-income artisans, traders, and drivers to college students, members of the armed forces, and government employees. Some of them were habitual clients; others paid only occasional visits. Commonly, the men engaged in a high rate of partner exchange, placing both themselves and their sexual contacts at high risk of contracting HIV. Apart from contact with the sex workers, the clients (approximately 60 per cent of whom were unmarried) reported intercourse with wives, girlfriends, and casual acquaintances.

Despite substantial progress being made to increase the women's knowledge about HIV and STIs, their clients still exhibit apathy and denial of the epidemic. A disturbing finding was that seropositive clients consistently denied being infected and refused to seek counselling. Assisting clients to educate themselves did not prove effective in the CRS programme. They remained unwilling to be identified or to assemble for education, and there were difficulties in finding a suitable forum and mode of communication. As a result, the programme's major strategy was to reinforce the initiatives and ingenuity of the women. For example, they used a poster from a taxi billboard campaign that read "No AIDS please, the family needs you," as a pointed reminder to clients of their obligation to protect their present and future families.

Condom Concerns

Consistent use of condoms has been considered the primary weapon for preventing HIV infection among sex workers as well as others who engage in risky behaviour. However, certain considerations need to be kept in mind when promoting condom use. The women have many reservations regarding the use of condoms. Some fear that they may retain the condoms in their vaginas, and others will not use condoms because they want to become pregnant. Some of the women were ignorant of the existence or benefits of condoms. Among the older sex workers, there is a belief that seminal fluid has nutritional value and contributes to good health when absorbed during intercourse. Men tend to regard the use of condoms as an alien practice that reduces sexual satisfaction and interferes with male control over the sexual relationship. And both groups are suspicious of potential sexual partners who want to use condoms, believing that they may have STIs.

When condom interventions were implemented in the CRS programme, the health and economic benefits were promoted by the staff. Women were educated about HIV, its modes of transmission, and the savings they would realize from using condoms regularly instead of having to buy expensive antibiotics (54 per cent of the women reported taking antibiotics daily). Within the first year of intervention, the number of commercial sex workers who never used condoms fell from 25 per cent to 3 per cent. The men still seemed reluctant to initiate condom use, however; in nearly all instances, the women reported that they had suggested and provided the condoms.

The lack of sufficient, affordable, and reliable supplies of quality condoms represents the single most pressing concern of condom-based interventions. Although a high degree of condom use has been achieved, the CRS programme suffered major setbacks because of unavailability. For example, the inadequate supply has made it impossible to meet more than one-third of the condom needs for the city of Calabar alone. The shortage has also curtailed the expansion of the programme to four additional cities for another two years. When no alternatives were available, poor-quality condoms were distributed for a three-month period in 1989. The frequent breakage severely discouraged condom use. Pursuing small supplies of condoms has become a major programme task, redirecting valuable time and energy away from other activities and contributing to the high rate of burnout among field-workers.

Looking Ahead

To forestall an onslaught of HIV infection and AIDS cases, immediate action is required. Nigeria must institute a series of comprehensive, prioritized programmes that take into account lessons learned from the experiences of other African countries where the epidemic has produced devastating repercussions.

The recent decision by government to integrate HIV prevention activities within the primary health-care system is an important step. But the system is still in its formative stages, and the time needed to implement this approach is not available in the battle to check the spread of HIV infection. Additional strategies—specifically, prevention initiatives that reach the entire population—are needed to supplement the longer-term programmes. And since only about 20 per cent of transfused blood is being tested for HIV, action must be taken to improve the security of the blood supply.

Commercial sex workers and their clients hold important keys to successful HIV prevention efforts. From the workers we can learn what intervention activities appeal to clients, who may be able to spread knowledge and positive attitudes to a larger base of men engaged in similar activities. We need to develop programmes for girls and women who are at an economic disadvantage and may be predisposed to enter the commercial sex industry. Programmes must also target women who are already working in the sex industry, as well as their clients.

Strategies for controlling HIV require careful thought and planning, and they must be sanctioned and supported by government as well as communities. This implies recognition of the practice of sex work and of the existence of girls and women who are on the verge of adopting this work as a livelihood.

In Nigeria, severe social and economic pressures have eroded cultural values and parental controls that normally would have a positive effect on HIV prevention. Many parents are unable to provide for and educate their daughters;

increasingly, they see the economic value of their daughters' sexuality as a potential source of support for the family. Girls desperate to support themselves and assist their families often migrate to urban areas in search of employment opportunities, and when that proves futile, they turn to sex work. Addressing the socioeconomic and cultural snares that offer young women no survival options besides sex work represents a major challenge for the future. Designing and implementing effective HIV-specific prevention programmes will become more complex because of the need to tailor efforts toward younger, more inexperienced, and less assertive women in the commercial sex industry. These programmes will have to identify specific strategies for sustaining the women's involvement in prevention activities.

The propensity of young men and women to engage in risky sexual behaviour is exacerbated by the absence of constructive sex education at home and in school. Traditionally, sex education was the work of aunts, grandparents, or other kin; many African parents still consider parental or school-based sex education a taboo. In urban settings, the traditionally appropriate relatives may not be available, yet teachers are not officially mandated to teach sex education in our schools. A culturally sensitive and appropriate sex-education curriculum needs to be developed and applied in schools. Parents and religious and community leaders must develop acceptable ways in which STI and HIV education can become an accepted theme for discussion.

Family-planning providers should orient their services toward birth and disease prevention to benefit those for whom unwanted pregnancies and STIs constitute major health risks. All women need to be empowered to initiate and adopt HIV prevention efforts. They should be provided with health services, education, and training to ensure other employment options, since the risk of HIV for full-time commercial sex workers with no other source of income is exceedingly high.

Comfort, a twenty-eight-year-old woman who "always" uses condoms, has recently become seropositive. She is a strong advocate of condom use among her peers, and her infection underscores the point that economic considerations supersede health concerns. When talking about condom use at a recent target-group workshop, she said, "It is easier to get a client to use a condom for his sex act, but when a man comes to stay overnight, you cannot get the same man to use condoms for each of many sex acts." A woman can earn five to six times more money from an all-night client. In the absence of alternative income options, the certainty of immediate monetary gain often takes priority over the potential risk of infection, even when the deadly nature of that risk is known.

Prevention-centred programmes in Nigeria, as elsewhere in Africa, are in dire need of more effective male-centred approaches. Modifying male attitudes about HIV and sexual behaviour is one of the significant factors in controlling this epidemic, and this constitutes a great challenge. But in confronting this epidemic, men also have a responsibility to respond by developing and championing male-focused activities and programmes that reflect relevant issues and appeal to their sensitivities.

Male responsibilities extend beyond their sexuality. Men hold privileged positions in government, society, community, and family. They possess the power and resources needed to ensure that initiatives also benefit women and young people. Prevention programmes that are spearheaded and supported at the highest level possible are urgently required in Nigeria. Our future is at stake.

10 Heading Off a Catastrophe

Mechai Viravaidya

Mechai Viravaidya is the founder and chairperson of the Population and Community Development Association of Thailand (PDA), a private, nonprofit family-planning and rural-development agency. An outspoken advocate for family planning, Viravaidya has become known for his use of humour in family-planning advocacy campaigns. He has been one of the nation's leading activists on the issues of HIV and AIDS and an early supporter of condom use for HIV prevention. He has served in numerous government positions, including senator, press spokesperson for the prime minister, and minister in the Office of the Prime Minster.

interviewed by Wasant Techawomgtham

Wasant Techawomgtham is a features writer for the Bangkok Post, *an English-language newspaper in Thailand. He has been reporting on HIV and AIDS issues for the past four years.*

I regard HIV not just as a health problem but as a societal problem. So long as there are no drugs to treat it and no vaccine to inoculate against it, there is only one thing we can do: take preventive measures. Since there is no effective treatment, we must care for people living with HIV and AIDS with compassion and respect for their human rights.

Prevention is the only cure. This is the key issue. There are three main factors in the Thai government's prevention programme: education, condoms, and the reduction of sexually transmitted infections (STIs).

We have launched an extensive education campaign that is included in school curricula from the primary level through the university. Education campaigns also focus on the workplace and rural areas. All five television stations and 485 radio stations throughout Thailand are now broadcasting a thirty-second spot every programme hour, with a focus on prevention and compassion. The prevention message tells people what HIV is, how it is contracted, how to prevent it, and what to do if they become HIV-positive. For example, people are urged not to have unprotected sex, and they are discouraged from patronizing the commercial sex trade. The compassion message is that anyone can contract HIV, that HIV is not contagious through everyday human contact, and that infected people have a place in our society and rights just like everyone else.

The second part of the prevention programme focuses on condoms. They have been used in Thailand for a long time. We have factories producing condoms for domestic use and for export. Supplies are available both from the government and from well over 130,000 stores. The problem is to ensure their use. Thai males' sexual behaviour is the primary factor in the spread of HIV. Men patronize sex workers and do not use condoms. The issue of cost is invalid, because if a man can pay for commercial sex, he can pay for condoms. We must ensure that people understand that they should reduce the number of sexual partners they have and use condoms whenever they have sex. At this time, men are the focal point of our education programmes.

The message on condoms is also being sent to the brothels, and we are trying to push them as hard as we can toward maximum use of condoms. The "100 per cent condom use" programme, a pilot project initiated in a few provinces, involves the governor, the provincial health office, the police, and operators of brothels. Brothel operators agree to allow the health office to conduct STI checks and blood tests for HIV on the women they employ. In return, they are allowed to conduct their business without police interference as long as no coercion is used on the women and no child prostitution is involved. If a brothel employee turns up with an STI, this indicates that condoms were not used. That brothel is penalized by being prevented from operating for one day. The second time an STI is diagnosed, the brothel is closed for a week, the third time, for a month. The fourth time this occurs, the brothel is closed permanently.

The third major aspect of our prevention campaign focuses on treating STIs. This is an important issue, because we know that STIs are a major factor in the transmission of HIV. People with STIs are much more susceptible to being infected with HIV. People have to be encouraged to get treatment, but they cannot be forced. The first thing we do is send out a general message to make people understand: "If you have an STI, your chances of contracting HIV are much higher. So come in, get treated, and use condoms to avoid any infection."

Sometimes people with STIs are unaware of the condition. Women are particularly vulnerable. Unlike their Western counterparts, Thai women do not go for medical checkups every six months or once a year, and some have never gone at all. We must get our message out simply, through women's magazines or even by inserting booklets inside sanitary-napkin boxes. The message must be clearly addressed to women, to let them know that they are at risk. A lot of them are going to contract STIs or HIV unknowingly from their husbands or boyfriends.

Our prevention programme must reach people in the rural areas as well as those in the cities. The government has already begun to reach down to the village level. Every province has an AIDS plan. Every workplace in the community, including the village committees, will be trained to provide information to people. At the same time, the importance of compassion and understanding must be stressed. We must remind others that we have people in our own villages who are infected and need to be taken care of. Chiefs, rural development officials, women's groups, health volunteers, private organization volunteers, monks, and teachers all must be taught to pass this message on.

I hope we leave no stone unturned. There are programmes geared toward the entire population, and some that are just for adults. Others are designed for specific groups in the workplace: vendors, construction workers, people working in gas stations, restaurant employees, and those who are self-employed or in the informal work sector. These workplace programmes are being administered by nongovernmental organizations (NGOs) in conjunction with local government agencies, the police, and the Ministry of Interior. We have programmes to educate university students who will then go out and teach the public. Our school programme focuses on children to prevent our problem from becoming worse in the future. HIV has been with us in Thailand for a long time, and we have to work with that in mind.

Prevention also requires addressing commercial sex work—both its demand and its supply. People continue to market and recruit young girls. There has been no effort to go to the villages and discourage girls from entering the sex trade. A recent study indicates that poverty is not the only thing that forces women into sex work. They are attracted by the consumerism and glamour that go with it—the glamour of having material possessions. Basically, education has a lot to do with it. Among all the commercial sex workers who have been interviewed, only 1 per cent have a secondary education. Girls with a secondary education have more employment options, so fewer are attracted to sex work.

Obviously, there is a need to provide alternative sources of income. I have gone to the business sector for help. The need is for specific training related to a product or a service for which there is a market or demand. This is going to be a long-term process. We also try to decentralize small factories; we have girls making shoes in the northeast as part of a subcontract with the Bata shoe factory.

These things are being done in many areas through the Thai Business Initiative in Rural Development (TBIRD) programme. In this programme, a company is asked to provide economic opportunities for the people of one village, so that there is no migration. The major emphasis is on young girls in the villages. Obviously, migration means migration to any job, including sex work. So far, sixty companies have cooperated. In these villages, not one girl has left to become a commercial sex worker, because we told them about HIV and provided them with alternative income. At our urging, people are even coming back to their villages.

Thai male sexual behaviour is key. If that does not change, we will have more HIV infection, which will have a great economic impact. There are basically three kinds of economic cost. The first is called forgone earnings—the income that is lost because infected people live shorter lives. An infected person, once he or she becomes ill, has to stop working. Once a person stops working, he or she stops receiving wages. Assume that each infected person will lose twenty-five years of his or her working life and that each person earns about $1,000 a year, which is lower than our per capita income. If we take into our calculation a social discount rate of 5 per cent, we lose about $17,200 of income for that person. Multiply that by the number of infected people to calculate the total income loss. The loss of income for each person is estimated to be about fifteen times the present per capita gross domestic product.

The second cost is that of health care, which we estimate to be about $1,000 per person per year. Again, this is a very conservative estimate. We assume that infected people will stay at home or in cheaper government hospitals rather than in private facilities. We also do not figure in the cost for expensive antiviral drugs such as AZT. Rough calculations indicate that the total annual health-care cost plus the value of lost income will grow from $100 million in 1991 to $2.2 billion by the year 2000. Over this ten-year period, we will probably lose about $8.7 billion due to HIV and related illnesses and death.

The third cost is the macroeconomic cost, including tourism, the export of labour, and the loss of prospective foreign investment. It will take time to calculate the total economic cost, but if all these costs are added up, the total is tremendous. Land prices will drop, as will tourism and labour exports.

The important point to consider is how much damage is likely to occur if we do not take action now. The sooner we slow the infection rate, the more manageable the situation becomes. For example, if 1993 were the peak year, the worst-case scenario is that we would have had more than 275,000 new HIV infections that year. This means that by 2001, the cumulative number of infected people would be more than 2 million. If we get serious in our prevention programme now, however, things may not be as bad as we think by the year 2001. But if we stand idly by and the infection rate peaks in 1997 instead, we will have 765,000 additional cases of HIV infection by the time 2001 rolls around.

The good thing about a projection like this is that once we identify the worst-case scenario, we can make another projection based on what we can do. For example, if we promote condom use, how many cases can we prevent? How many more if we tackle the STI situation? If we stay on course, we will still have a problem, but it will no longer be a catastrophe.

We can probably prevent 600,000 cases from the cumulative number of more than 2 million originally projected for the year 2001. This is a 30 per cent reduction.

Right now, we have about 80,000 hospital beds, and they are not enough. If nothing is done and we leave the situation to continue as it is, in the year 2000, we will have about 180,000 people diagnosed with AIDS and 160,000 deaths that year. That 180,000 is already more than double the number of beds in our hospitals. What we need is a home-based care system in which people with HIV-related illnesses can spend a couple of days each month in a hospital as necessary and the rest of their time at home. Then the community and family could take care of each other with the assistance of mobile doctors. The Ministry of Public Health and all universities with medical schools have had meetings to plan an ambulatory home-based care system. Obviously, extended families will have to give care. This is why 50 per cent of our campaign focuses on compassion. Whenever there is no family left or the family cannot help, the Buddhist temples would become places of solace and could be used as orphanages in the future.

It is always daunting to examine how much money must be spent. However, it is even more daunting to look at how much money will be lost if we do not begin prevention now. Investing in prevention programmes makes economic sense. Luckily, our mass media are owned by the government; otherwise, the half-minute HIV educational messages would cost approximately $48 million. Government personnel who are involved in the educational programming are already paid for. Companies participate in programmes on their own time and use their own resources. We have estimated that the cost of the programme in kind and in cash for 1991 came to about $112 million.

HIV has done damage here as it has in every other country. Whether the damage can be contained depends very much on the leadership. We have to follow through on our campaign. We must be vigilant. If people are seriously involved, it will put pressure on the government to pay attention. We cannot sit back and wait for the government to set the direction. As a private citizen, I campaigned until the government had to respond. We cannot assume that the government will think for itself. Currently, we have good leadership on this issue, but if the next government is not concerned, we will have to push from the outside to force it to address the epidemic. Otherwise, we will all pay a price we cannot afford.

11   We Are Our Own Worst Enemies

Godfrey Sealey

Godfrey Sealey is a playwright and HIV activist living in Trinidad and Tobago. He wrote the first Caribbean play about AIDS, One of Our Sons Is Missing. *His* AIDA, the Wicked Wench of the World, *a pantomime in the carnival genre addressing HIV and discrimination, was performed at the Fifth International Conference on AIDS in Montreal in 1989.*

During the early part of the last decade, when the world was just beginning to wake up to the threat of HIV, we in Trinidad were in the later stages of an oil boom. As one politician proudly announced, money was not a problem for our nation, and neither was anything else, it seemed. When the first cases of AIDS were diagnosed here in 1983, all were among gay men, and everyone, including other gays, assumed that this was just an obscure disease that would not affect them. We all believed that the good times of the oil boom were here to stay, and in the midst of this euphoria, society became slightly more tolerant toward homosexuals. Because homosexuality was, and still is, against the law, homosexuals were discreet about their social interaction. But even though the gay scene was not public, there was always something going on. We had gay nightclubs in Port of Spain, and there were frequent private parties where homosexuals could socialize freely.

As long as a person does not flaunt his or her sexual orientation, society will usually ignore what is not considered the norm, but the pressure to convert or conform, though often subtle, is unremitting. In Trinidad, even in the best of times, homosexuality is looked upon as an abomination. Anyone considered to be so inclined is condemned as a sinner of the highest order. Gay persons, when confronted, are often asked whether they believe in God. The hope is that the answer will be no, because that would supply sufficient reason for their homosexuality. Regardless of the answer, a campaign will be launched to save them. The Bible is quoted, religious literature and prayer are offered, and they are urged to attend church. These attempts at conversion are so intense that many people succumb, sometimes temporarily, in fear of ostracism from peers and under threat of eternal damnation.

Our society is so homophobic that openness and honesty about one's sexuality can lead to victimization on the job or being expelled from the home. In our society, most unmarried young people live with their parents. In some instances, gays have even had their lives threatened by their own parents.

Human sexuality is not a topic that is discussed publicly in this society. As children, we were never taught about sex by our parents or our teachers; most of us learned from books, films, and conversations with others, or by experimenting. As a result, many adults are unable to fully express themselves sexually without feeling guilty or risking censure. People do not explore the potential of lovemaking. The prime focus of sex, more often than not, is penetration. Gays rarely have a true understanding of their sexual orientation and do not assert themselves. Instead, homosexuality remains unaccepted by society and is not deemed a serious issue that should be addressed.

It should not be surprising then that gays in Trinidad consider themselves to be second-class citizens. They inflict this added burden on themselves because of a belief that they must make amends for their perceived inadequacy. Many gay people think that their homosexuality is temporary and that they will change once it is time to settle down and have children. Regardless of how often their settling down is postponed, the idea that they will not always be like this remains.

An example comes to mind: I was speaking to a friend who has sexual relationships with men. Normally he keeps a very low profile, but these activities occur during carnival, the one time he allows himself the freedom of sexual expression. While talking about what he desired from life, he labelled the desires he has for men a slackness, a vice. In spite of his pleasurable experiences, he declared his intention to reform and take on "the responsibility of a man" by the year's end. He believed that his homosexuality was immature behaviour and that heterosexual activity was part of his coming of age.

It is in the midst of this climate of ignorance, ambivalence, misinformation, guilt, self-delusion, homophobia, and intrigue that gay people try to survive. Given their fear of becoming pariahs and the general reluctance of Trinidadians to discuss sexual behaviour, it is little wonder that even in the face of HIV, gays are reluctant to step forward to address the issue. Instead they remain silent, in spite of the fact that many of those dying from the disease here are homosexuals.

In recent years, I have seen what this silence, denial, and fear have done to friends. I have watched people deny their sexuality. I have witnessed many friends who were dying of HIV-related illnesses refuse to acknowledge that they had the disease and refuse offers of support and assistance. This denial often places us in the untenable position of remaining silent while knowing that their friends and families are uninformed of their own exposure to the disease. Out of respect for their privacy, I have changed their names in the stories that follow.

A few years ago, a friend who had always been fat started to lose weight. He claimed to be dieting, but after noticing some dark spots on his arms and his upper body, I began to question him. Bill, who was a psychiatric nurse, brushed my questions aside, annoyed that I would challenge his medical expertise. He continued to lose weight but still refused to discuss his health. Weeks later he telephoned my lover and asked him to visit; even then, all he said was that he was contemplating suicide. Bill died in the hospital a few days later, alone, and still in possession of his secret. His burial arrangements were handled in silence, and no one knew where or when his funeral took place. To the best of my knowledge, he never informed any of his former partners of their exposure to HIV.

When rumours began to circulate that Paul, an old schoolmate, had AIDS, he withdrew from all social activity. I visited him to offer my advice and support, but he steadfastly denied any illness. Months passed and I heard nothing from or about Paul. I attempted to find him, but no one seemed to know where he was. After an extensive search, I finally located him in the hospital. When Paul died, his friends wondered if they could have done more, but he had chosen to allow the virus to take control of his life and refused our offers of support.

Too often the threat of public disclosure is more frightening than the disease itself. John had always been a popular person on the gay scene. He was affectionately referred to as "Mother" and had a reputation for hosting many vibrant parties. When John started to lose weight and gradually began growing weak, I became concerned about my friend's health. I thought that he would be honest with me, but unfortunately, I was mistaken. Because of his fear that disclosure would lead to scandal, John concocted a story to lead people off the track. Suddenly he claimed that he had a history of lung problems. When that was insufficient, he furnished what was purported to be a medical report proving that he was not HIV-positive. In spite of numerous attempts to assist him, he refused to budge and died without ever admitting that he had AIDS.

As distressing as I found John's attitude to be, what happened when a dear friend of mine became ill was far more disturbing. We had known each other for years, and I truly cherished his friendship. We worked in the theater together. In fact, he was the person who had christened me with a stage name that has stuck to this day. Tim was a professional window dresser and costume designer. He was a very talented young man with a bright future ahead of him. Tim and his lover Joe had been together for a number of years. The fact that Joe had a wife and children did not seem to hamper the relationship. To avoid suspicion and give the impression that he was straight, Tim began to dissociate himself from his previous circle of friends and developed a relationship with a woman. We spoke on numerous occasions about his relationships with Joe and with his girlfriend. Whenever the subject of HIV arose, Tim, who was paranoid about the disease, refused to discuss it.

After months without any communication between us, Tim telephoned me. He said that he had been losing weight for no particular reason and was very worried. I think he was most afraid that his new circle of straight friends would suspect that he might have contracted HIV and begin to question his sexuality. During our conversation, I suggested that he get tested for HIV, but Tim was not prepared to do that at the time. He said that he would telephone me if he had a change of heart or needed some advice. Then Tim told me that his girlfriend was pregnant.

For weeks I heard nothing from him. Months later, when I found out that Tim was bedridden, I visited him immediately. When I saw him I could not believe my eyes. He was in the terminal stage of the illness and had already been hospitalized. His girlfriend, who had recently given birth, visited him daily but was uninformed about the true nature of his condition.

During the earlier stages, Tim had insinuated that he suffered from a "spirit lash," an evil curse that had been cast upon him by an enemy. His mother, who held very strong spiritual beliefs, took the bait and tried to find spiritual cures for her son's ailments. When she realized that none of these cures was working, the ultimate solution was indeed hospitalization. Tim's girlfriend did not believe the spirit lash story and waited to find out the truth. The truth, however, was never revealed. Tim went to his grave never having spoken to her about his sexual orientation, his previous lifestyle, or Joe being his lover. To this day, she knows nothing and continues to be friendly with Joe.

After Tim's death, everything seemed to return to normal. I did not pursue the issues surrounding Tim's death because I believed that it was Joe's responsibility to inform both his wife and Tim's girlfriend about their exposure to the disease. Though I am very concerned about the welfare of both women, I have not spoken with Joe to address the ethics of the situation, but I intend to do so soon. I know that Joe does not wish to admit that he had a sexual affair with a man and that such a disclosure, in his mind, far outweighs the dangers of HIV.

Ours is a country where silence and denial are preferable because they keep scandal and confusion at bay. Knowing this, I would not be surprised if Joe's wife either refused to believe his confession or brushed the issue off. She might tell Joe not to tell anyone and reassure him that everything is all right. Like many other women, she may reject her husband's homosexuality or bisexuality, and she will assume that her womanhood will convert him to heterosexuality.

At a party a few months ago, I was talking to a friend who had been experiencing chest pains recently. I am certain that he is HIV-positive, but he will not entertain the thought. We began to discuss his love life, and he informed me that he was having an affair with a married man. We talked about sex, and he eventually told me that his partner does not like to use condoms. I reminded him that a condom was necessary to protect against the transmission of HIV, but he refused to believe that there was a reason for him to practice safer sexual relations. As far as he was concerned, because the man was married and not active on the gay scene, this meant that he must be "clean."

I found his attitude quite disturbing and indeed very selfish. Not only was my friend deluding himself about his lover's prior sexual contacts, but he was not taking his own sexual history into account and considering the possible danger that he might pose to his lover and his lover's wife. In fact, he claimed that they were in love and had nothing to worry about, as if it were true that love conquers all.

People are so insecure about their sexual orientation that they will go to absurd lengths to prove that they are not what others think they are, regardless of whether it is true or not. They are constantly hiding behind masks, trying to fit into a society that abhors homosexuality. They lie to themselves and believe that by working doubly hard, by overcompensating, they will be loved and respected just like any other member of our society. To avoid being ridiculed, some try whenever possible to associate with heterosexuals.

When HIV first appeared and seemed to be affecting only homosexuals, it was popularly assumed to be a curse from God sent to eradicate an evil from the world. The police, who had long maintained a vendetta against gays, used the advent of HIV as justification for reinforcing long-standing prejudices. As a result, local parks that served as meeting places for homosexuals, especially the poor, are now closed at night. Men found in the park after hours have been harassed or beaten by the police. Many gays feel helpless to take recourse against this behaviour, so there is little outcry.

Current public education efforts are focused exclusively on the heterosexual segment of society. Information that is relevant to the needs of gay men must be disseminated, but because of the stigma attached to homosexuality, there has been a great deal of procrastination on the part of the authorities. Homosexuals need to know that isolation is unnecessary and that there are people who are concerned about their well-being.

Although HIV focus-group sessions have been organized by nongovernmental organizations to fulfil the needs of homosexuals in this country, the government is doing little to follow up on these sessions. Intense homophobia and the fear of appearing to condone homosexuality have prevented the National AIDS Programme from creating desperately needed information for the gay community. As a result, the responsibility of providing information to gays has been taken on by a few individuals, who must constantly monitor the actions of the National AIDS Programme.

The only information available to homosexuals is via word of mouth, the HIV clinic, and the national AIDS hotline. But very few persons, gay or heterosexual, seek or properly use these sources. Instead, most persons who have contracted HIV, especially gay people, prefer to remain silent about their health. Even when gay men go to the clinic, many refuse to identify themselves as homosexuals, so the information they receive is not always relevant to their lifestyles. Gays who telephone the hotline follow a similar pattern, asking questions in a roundabout fashion rather than identifying their specific needs.

In communities where spirituality plays a major role in the lives of the population, it is uncertain what effect prevention programmes will have. Many leave their problems to the will of God or rely on visions for curing illnesses. In a country like ours, where there is no organized treatment programme, people consider themselves fortunate to have such alternatives.

Another problem is that people do not easily discuss their sexual habits, particularly if they are from a middle-class background. The gay community in Trinidad and Tobago, as in nearly every other community in this part of the world, operates as part of a larger, strict class structure. Middle-class gays generally avoid associating with gays from the lower class. To some extent, HIV in Trinidad has served to deepen class divisions, because the majority of those dying from HIV-related illnesses are working-class or poor gay men. As a result, people tend to associate the disease with the lower economic class and their supposedly wanton sexual habits. Many upper-class gays believe that HIV happens only to "them," the drag queens and boys who meet one another in the parks.

Getting gays to consider themselves first-class citizens has become an even tougher task now that HIV and AIDS are a reality. Attempts have been made, by a few homosexuals, to make gay people more conscious not only of their rights but of the virus and the disease as well. These individuals have taken on the task of educating others about responsible sexual relationships and safer sex practices, and they are also providing information about the disease. To prevent HIV transmission, condoms are distributed at parties, but there is still too much resistance to change. Some complain about condoms, claiming that they are uncomfortable, that they break, or that they diminish sexual satisfaction. Others believe that because they do not have sex with popular people, they are safe. They truly believe that they do not need to use condoms because they know their partners. Macho gays think that they are invulnerable to HIV.

The ill and dying are faceless: we do not know who they are, and society does not seem to care. When death strikes someone from the middle or upper class, people are told that he succumbed to a more acceptable disease that he had been suffering from for years. Other people just seem to disappear; sometimes one hears that they moved without leaving a forwarding address. If it is public knowledge that a gay man died of AIDS, he is buried with little or no respect. The unsolemn affair is usually a hurried cremation that is done secretly to avoid publicity.

At the heart of the lack of response to the epidemic by Trinidad's already fragile and fragmented small gay community is a sense of helplessness. HIV caught them unawares, and they were not prepared to take any action against it. Lacking reliable information sources about the disease, many concluded that the only solution was to completely withdraw from the gay scene, or at least appear to do so. HIV was looked upon as something shameful and subject to ridicule, and anyone suspected of being infected with the virus was immediately scorned. This has become a popular tactic to divert suspicion away from those doing the ridiculing.

In what has been a recurring pattern among homosexuals, many believe that they must expose others in order to protect themselves. The sad fact is that many of us do not trust one another, and this is why we have not become a true unified community. In the best of times, this creates an environment of deception and self-delusion, but with the advent of HIV in Trinidad and Tobago, it becomes a deadly crisis. Gays are not represented on the national level. If we do not organize into a cohesive group with common goals, issues relating to our lives and survival in the face of HIV will not be addressed by government or society.

Many go to great lengths to dissociate themselves from anyone even vaguely suspected of being HIV-positive. Public gatherings of homosexuals have become less frequent. People have shown little or no compassion for their peers who are living with HIV, reflecting a morbid fear of the disease itself and an even greater fear of being exposed as a homosexual. This paranoia is so extreme that many have refused to visit their closest friends who have been diagnosed with AIDS. Those who are dying of the illness often deny, even to their closest friends, that they are infected. Ironically, many blame themselves for becoming infected and see HIV as their punishment.

Their fear of being discovered has prompted many gays with HIV to concoct the most harebrained stories to divert suspicion. Thus the blame is directed away from the infected person, and there is no more nasty business about homosexuality and HIV. Unfortunately, this scenario only hides the problems that we must identify and acknowledge in order to confront HIV rationally.

Gays have been trying to foster monogamous unions, and couples often use condoms in the early stages of their relationship. But as their love deepens, the resolve to use condoms diminishes. When lovers are comfortable with each other, the assumption is that there is no need to worry. The possibility of HIV infection is obscured by the pleasures of romantic love.

Obviously, programmes are needed that inform the gay community about HIV and its prevention. What is needed most of all, though, is a sense of unity and a greater understanding of ourselves and our sexuality. I hope that in the near future the gay community sees fit to demand adequate information and treatment and realizes the need for unification in the battle for self-acceptance and respect from society at large. We have to realize that we are our own best support. This is going to be a difficult task, but unless it is achieved, we will end up being key contributors to our own self-destruction. Unless people begin to acknowledge their sexuality and behaviour openly, they will put ever-increasing numbers of others at risk.

12 The Disease That Dares Not Say Its Name

Omari Haruna Kokole

Omari Haruna Kokole is the associate director of global cultural studies at the State University of New York at Binghamton. Kokole received his Ph.D. in political science from Dalhousie University in Canada. He is the author of Dimensions of Africa's International Relations.

"Out there somewhere, alone and frightened." So sang my compatriot Philly Bongoley Lutaaya, describing how it felt to be a person living with HIV. Lutaaya, one of Uganda's most famous entertainers, began speaking about living with HIV in 1989. He was the first well-known Ugandan to publicly acknowledge that he was infected. His struggle during the last few months of his life to raise Uganda's public awareness of the epidemic became the subject of a moving documentary, *Born in Africa*. Given the stigma surrounding the disease and the tendency for society to ostracize persons with HIV, Lutaaya's was a bold and selfless act. His public stance and subsequent death warned those who cared to listen that unless they took the necessary precautions, this could also happen to them.

When I first heard Lutaaya sing "Out there somewhere, alone and frightened," the song moved me, although the lyrics had no immediate or personal meaning. A few months later, I began to understand what Lutaaya must have experienced when he first learned of his condition. This essay is partly about the late Lutaaya, partly about myself, and partly about one of my sisters: three Ugandan nationals, relatively young adults in our twenties and thirties, whose lives have been fundamentally affected by this deadly global epidemic. Lutaaya died as a result of his infection with HIV. I once faced the possibility of being infected with HIV and found myself wrestling with the knowledge that I might die as a result. Yakanye, one of my three sisters, tested positive for HIV and now manifests some symptoms of AIDS.

I have not lived in Uganda since 1976, but like many of my fellow Ugandan expatriates, I knew of a few friends back home who had died from HIV-related illnesses. I also knew how widespread the epidemic had become. I occasionally visited the country, and I knew theoretically that I was as vulnerable as my late musician compatriot and others had been. But I lulled myself into believing that HIV happened to other people, not to me.

In the spring of 1990, I spent some time at home in Uganda. Not long after I returned to the United States, I went for a complete physical examination, my first in three years. After two consecutive tests indicated that my white-blood-cell count was below normal, the doctor made it clear that there was reason for concern. He suggested that we examine all possibilities, including cancer and HIV, and suggested that I consider being tested for the virus.

My response was that if I had contracted HIV, I preferred not to know. I thought of the disease as a death sentence. To know would be to deny myself the luxury of a normal life from that moment on. Instead, I would be obsessed with the idea of imminent death, and this would colour and influence each and every act, thought, and feeling of mine until my dying day. It would be sheer agony, and I was not sure that I could withstand such an ordeal. Evidently my attitude was shared by others, because I have since heard it said that most people in Kampala (Uganda's capital) who donate blood do not want to know the results.

In response, my doctor reminded me that I was still healthy and that if I did test positive for HIV, there was a good chance of prolonging my life by protecting me from the opportunistic infections that are often a part of this disease. Apprehensively, I agreed to be tested. My blood sample was taken, and I was told that the results would arrive in two weeks. The subsequent fourteen days were the longest, toughest days I have ever lived.

I hesitated to confide in others, partly because I feared I would be harshly judged and ostracized. Thus, having resolved not to confide in anyone that I had been tested and was awaiting the decisive results, loneliness was the most painful part of my ordeal. The words of that Philly Lutaaya song took on an immediacy and resonance greater than I had ever imagined possible.

Throughout that terrible waiting period, I kept wondering, what if the results turn out to be positive? I knew of two friends, former classmates at Makerere University in Uganda, who had died of HIV-related illnesses in the 1980s. They, in turn, had other relatives and friends who had succumbed. Was I going to die young, in my thirties, like Philly, John, Margaret, and Susan? Kampala has been described as a place where "a roadside coffin maker says he sells more of his product for burying young adults than the elderly." How much time was left before one of these coffins would be purchased for me? As I pondered my future in the face of HIV, there was also some anger: what had I done to deserve this fate?

During that long, lonely waiting period, I wondered about the broader meaning and repercussions of my death. I am the first and only member of my family to attend university. My ethnic group in Uganda, the Kakwa, constitutes a small community. We were scattered three ways by European colonialism when the artificial boundaries were drawn; other Kakwa are nationals of Zaire and the Sudan. Now HIV threatens to eliminate our small ethnic group and preempt the fruits of my people's achievements.

In Africa, the economically productive are more likely to be infected with HIV. The disease tends to strike young adults, those most likely to leave behind children and dependents. As a result, premature death carries, among other things, serious economic, political, psychological, and sociological consequences.

The late Philly Lutaaya was survived by four young children. My two teenage daughters remained in Africa when I left to pursue my graduate education overseas. Both Apayi and Amori were attending school in Kenya. I was responsible for funding their education and for providing virtually all their material needs. As the cloud of HIV hung over my head that summer, I thought about what would happen to my daughters if the test results were positive and if I were to die in the next few years. Because of extended family obligations, I had not saved enough money to ensure that they could complete their education. Should I look for a guardian or prospective sponsor for my daughters? How and when would I break the news to them? Should I warn them about the danger of Daddy's fate befalling them? After all, the two girls were teenagers and vulnerable to the virus.

I worried too about my parents and other siblings. After my death, who would help them financially? The political anarchy and turmoil in Uganda since the 1970s had scattered my family. My father was a refugee in Zaire. Having witnessed wanton lawlessness and violence in Uganda, he swore never to return. My mother only recently returned to Uganda from the Sudan. Both my parents were more or less my dependents.

Two of my siblings, though not completely dependent on me, were partially my wards. Then there were members of the wider extended family who looked to me for help from time to time.

Dr. Sam I. Okware, Uganda's deputy director of medical services, was not overstating when he said, "Here, nobody is born an individual. If an important person dies, it is not one individual dying; it is a community." As the man who paid the school fees for almost all the children of his home village, Dr. Okware's obligations were much heavier than mine. But in a sense, he was speaking for many of us when he remarked, sadly, "If I go, the whole village is gone."

The two-week waiting period for the results of my HIV test ended on a Monday. Early that morning my telephone rang. It was my doctor saying, "Dr. Kokole. I have some good news for you. You are HIV-free."

What a relief! I felt as if a ton of bricks had been lifted off my back, even though my doctor advised that I take another blood test to ensure that I was also cancer-free. But psychologically, HIV was the more terrifying prospect. Maybe it had to do with society's contrasting responses to the two conditions. If I had cancer, I would be less ostracized, less stigmatized than if I had HIV. Fortunately, the results from that blood test were available the following day. Again I received good news.

And yet my feelings of elation and relief were tinged with sorrow, for my sister had not been as lucky. When I saw Yakanye in Kampala in May 1990, I knew that she had not been feeling well for some time. Although the thought occurred to me that she might have contracted HIV, it did not register as a distinct possibility, because she did not look ill or emaciated. I was devastated the afternoon that Yakanye came to my hotel and told me that she had been tested and that the results were positive. I love my sister deeply, and I tried to respond sympathetically and calmly. I did not ask her how she might have caught the virus. To do so would have looked as if I were trying to apportion blame. Yakanye was in enough pain already, and I did not want to add to it. Besides, how she contracted HIV was not the issue. Now that we knew she had it, what were we going to do about it? The documentary about Philly Lutaaya contributed to my enlightened response to this family crisis.

I told Yakanye not to worry too much and encouraged her to continue with her education. I reminded her that doctors and scientists continue to work very hard at finding a cure, and that it was possible one would be found soon. I urged her to seek support and counselling and continue to do so after my return to the United States. I succeeded in persuading Yakanye to join several support groups, including The AIDS Support Organization (TASO), founded by Noerine Kaleeba. But despite my external calm, I was deeply shaken. I began to think of how to reconcile myself to the reality that she might not be alive for much longer, that she might die in her late twenties.

Had my sister's condition developed after, rather than before, my own scare, my initial response to her tragedy would have been different. Rather than pretending not to be worried and sad, I would have helped her confront and deal with these very painful and unavoidable emotions. After my experience, I promptly wrote to Yakanye about what I had gone through. I told her that as a result, I now had a deeper and more compassionate understanding of her situation. I apologized for not having cared enough about her fate. Much to my surprise and reassurance, she responded by saying that she always knew I cared and was sure that I genuinely shared her anguish. My admiration for my sister's courage and perseverance and her capacity to retain her sanity in such personally tragic and trying circumstances knows no bounds. The fact that Yakanye gave me permission to share her news with anyone of my choosing is but one example of her courage.

Given how scared I was during those critical weeks of waiting, my better understanding now extends to what so many others are facing, and my admiration has grown for those who test positive for HIV and are strong enough not to go crazy afterward. I respect their fortitude and perseverance because, for so many people, living with HIV must be terribly difficult and very solitary. Those of us who are HIV-free should relate to people who are infected with greater compassion and understanding. In the ultimate analysis, HIV is our collective disease.

Within the family, I have persuaded other members to respond positively and supportively to Yakanye. As the eldest offspring and son, my role has been helped by tradition, which respects age and seniority. But while I anxiously awaited my test results, I could not help but wonder how the news that both my sister and I were HIV-positive would affect the family. Difficult as it is for a family to discover that one among them has this disease, think how much greater the tragedy is when two or more of its members are stricken. In many parts of Uganda, the broader implications of such intrafamilial catastrophes are very serious.

One is reminded of Beatrice Habeenzy of Hamuntamba, Zambia, who left her husband because she believed that he had transmitted HIV to her. Beatrice has lost one child already, and her nursing baby may also be infected. Noerine Kaleeba's husband died of HIV-related illnesses. Of her two sisters who have been diagnosed with AIDS, one is now dead. She says that her family is not unusual. Then there is the sixty-eight-year-old woman near the Ugandan town of Masaka who has lost three of her four children to AIDS. She now lives with her one remaining son and twenty-eight grandchildren, some of whom probably carry the virus too.

HIV has already affected the lives of countless people in many countries, both directly and indirectly. As the epidemic grows, the situation can only get worse. The emotional, economic, social, and political toll is already enormous and is unlikely to diminish unless a cure or vaccine for the virus is discovered before the end of this century.

Health and development are intimately related. A society with vast numbers of ill members cannot be productive enough to develop itself. Now, along with the health, economic, and development problems Africa already has, HIV has arrived with a bang. Like most developing countries, Uganda already had several killer diseases before the advent of HIV. However, because the virus is targeting the most productive members and the future leaders of society, its full impact differs radically from that of most other fatal diseases already challenging developing countries.

The political turmoil and violence in Uganda have had a staggering economic cost. Uganda's productive capacity diminished greatly as its modest infrastructure was neglected or, worse, demolished. In time, the economy fared so badly that the term *salary* became meaningless. For example, a professor at Makerere University earns less than the equivalent of U.S. $50 a month, with approximately the same purchasing power.

The African continent has lost many skilled and educated young people to the brain drain. Now, in Uganda and in other countries, HIV threatens those who chose to remain. The loss of these "stayees," as they are called, can only exacerbate the problems of an already ailing economy and dislocated society.

Most African countries do not yet have free elementary education. Indeed, for most parents, it is costly to educate a child. Without the support provided by other educated or affluent members of the family or village, many children would never be able to attend school. The termination of such support because of HIV and the burdening of elderly grandparents have alarming implications for the future.

In 1990, the population of the Republic of Uganda was estimated at approximately 17.5 million and was expected to surpass the 30 million mark by the year 2015. If the epidemic continues to grow at its present speed, however, by 2015, Uganda is likely to have a population of only 20 million. Superficially, this would appear to be good news, because much of the developing world is endangered by population growth rates that surpass economic growth and performance rates. But this 10 million shortfall in population will comprise those young, economically active people who have died of HIV-related illnesses as well as those who will never be born as a consequence of HIV. Meanwhile, it is estimated that by 2010, between 5 and 6 million Ugandan children will be parentless. The numbers of grandparents who will be raising their grandchildren, and burying their own children will continue to increase. This situation imperils many of the elderly economically, for they no longer have anyone to provide for them in their old age. Placing the burden for the survival of young children on their fragile shoulders increases the children's vulnerability as well.

Uganda already has hundreds of thousands of parentless children as a result of its civil wars and violent politics. If projections for the future are accurate, the HIV epidemic will significantly swell that subpopulation. These children are likely to be underfed, underschooled, underhoused, and generally under-cared-for. Ultimately, they are likely to be less than fully integrated, productive members of society. The indigenous extended-family system is already burdened by the effects and side effects of civil wars, rural-urban migration, and economic dislocation, among many other factors. It simply cannot be expected to cope with new and unprecedented demands. For a country that has already experienced so much turbulence and bloodletting, HIV endangers its economy, stability, and morale.

Many indigenous customs and traditions are likely to be severely tested. Already there is evidence that mourning periods and funerals are becoming shorter. It is also likely that many Ugandans will not feel guilty about failing to meet the inordinately heavy and growing extended-family obligations created by the epidemic. All this adds up to future crises in an already troubled country. The cumulative, long-term impact and implications of the epidemic for African countries are mind-boggling. It is impossible to calculate the damage, havoc, and anguish HIV will generate in Africa and, indeed, worldwide. But there is little doubt that the bottom line will be substantial.

In Africa, HIV has an urban bias. But because the rural-urban connection on the continent is more of a continuum and less of a dichotomy, it is hardly surprising that the virus has begun to make inroads into the rural areas as well. The vast majority of Africans reside in rural areas and, because of the constant traffic between town and village, the virus seems to be headed in that direction.

The future looks grim, and the widespread tendency not to be completely open about HIV can only exacerbate the situation. Regardless of their reasons, governments in Africa and elsewhere that attempt to minimize or conceal the presence of the disease in their countries are wrong. To behave as if HIV were not a reality—and a raging and growing one at that—is ultimately much more dangerous than confronting it and working to do something about it. Governments as well as private individuals must face HIV head-on.

It is clear that prevailing negative and counterproductive attitudes will be difficult—but not impossible—to change. In order for this to occur, governments must be committed to frank discussions and the investment of more energy and resources for public education programmes and mass media efforts. Society must face up to the fact that HIV is a real disease that strikes real human beings such as you and me, and unless we confront its reality, we are all endangered.

13 The Power to Silence Us

Aimée Mwadi

> *Aimée Mwadi works with the Institut National de Reserches Biomedicales in Zaire. She was trained at the University of Kinshasa Faculty of Medicine and the Institut Pasteur in France. She was chairperson of the Society for Women Against AIDS in Zaire.*

The story I am going to tell you is true. I have loved, and perhaps I have betrayed. I now have the peace of mind I need to write and convey the depths of my feelings. I carry the weight not only of the years but also of what was unsaid and everything that was hidden.

I married when I was nineteen years old; now I am the mother of three boys. Our home in Zaire was a modest one, and we were full of love for each other. However, as time passed, I became increasingly insecure because my husband did not allow me to express myself or to have basic rights as an individual. I decided to continue my education, despite his disapproval. After I completed my university studies, I had the good fortune to go to France to train as a specialist in HIV diagnostic research techniques. Upon my return, my husband announced that he was officially a polygamist and planned to have as many wives as he could afford. I did not become jealous, but rather indignant and scornful. This was not the first time that I had been faced with his infidelity, so I was not surprised.

I was defenseless and had no one to confide in. Even my mother could not be my confidante, because I could not discuss the ideas that were beginning to form in my mind. In our culture, out of respect for our elders, we do not discuss sexual problems with our parents. Given the seriousness of my problem, I almost dared to confide in her, but I held back because I believed that her response would be quite different from mine.

I spent days absorbed in thought and inner conflict. I weighed the negative and positive consequences of my decision. Finally I regained my bearings because of a recurring thought: this is a matter of life and death. With this in mind, I gathered the courage to begin an open dialogue with my husband. Since he had informed me of his polygamous intentions, we had not been speaking; our children had been serving as our intermediaries.

During our first conversation, I asked him a number of questions, including whether he knew his partners' HIV status and their sexual behaviour. His response was that this issue was of little importance because HIV did not exist in the town where he lived. I tried to make him understand that the large cities were not the only places affected by HIV; HIV threatened rural areas as well. I even used statistical data to support my position regarding the HIV situation in our country. I also tried to dispel the widespread myth that HIV was an imaginary syndrome invented to discourage sexual activity. (SIDA, the acronym for AIDS in French, is believed to represent Syndrome Imaginaire pour Decourager L'Amour.)

Other tactics that I employed included reminding my husband that the future of our sons depended on our remaining healthy and productive. Unfortunately, he remained firm in his resolve to practice polygamy and refused to change his decision. It was upon this refusal that I demanded that he either have an HIV test or use condoms if he wanted to continue to have sexual relations with me. He rejected both requests, and that was the beginning of our duel. He tried many things to change my mind—blackmail, threats, and sometimes physical abuse—but I stood by my decision to protect myself and my children from his high-risk sexual behaviour.

My husband commenced his polygamous practices and returned to our home every three months for one-week visits. When he realized that I remained as determined as ever, he assembled some members of his family to inform them of my disobedience. But he could not state the cause of my behaviour openly or explain our true problem, because in Africa, couples cannot discuss problems regarding their intimate lives in public.

During this time, the laboratory where I worked was the best equipped in the field of virology, particularly in HIV research and diagnosis. We treated patients from throughout the country as well as citizens of neighbouring countries. It was frightening. People who looked healthy were HIV-positive. The high mortality rate left us in a state of shock. Of particular interest to me was the predicament of women and parentless children. Thus, living the reality of HIV at work encouraged me to take the situation in my personal life very seriously.

I often wondered whether I had made the right decision. I asked myself whether I was suffering from HIV-related phobia. But in spite of the constraints, arguments, threats, and false accusations of infidelity made by my husband's family, I remained firm in my decision. I thought of leaving my home, but concern about my children's future kept me from doing so, especially now that their father had rejected us.

Finally my husband spoke openly with his brothers about our conflict. They held a family meeting to decide what punishment they would impose on me for humiliating their brother. There were endless arguments between my husband and me, and often, for no reason, he ordered me to leave the house. Sometimes my sisters-in-law would visit, endlessly repeating that their mother had not given birth to their brother for me exclusively. They said that my jealousy was like an electric current and that one day it would electrocute me. I spent two years in this atmosphere, and as a result, my health suffered terribly. My husband officially left me in August 1988. I saw him again three years later when he appeared before the court; I had begun divorce proceedings against him for moral and material abandonment.

In 1989, I cofounded a branch of the Society for Women and AIDS in Africa (SWAA). I am now the national president. This has been an opportunity for me to meet with women from all walks of life to discuss our views on the HIV epidemic as it affects women. Through my personal experience and the experiences of others, I learned that many women suffer in silence. We have been educated to respect the African tradition of resignation: a wife is at the service of her husband and his family. If we only knew how many of our sisters have been sent to the hereafter by the very resignation that our grandmothers and mothers taught and continue to teach us. Now HIV has changed many aspects of our lives, and humanity is facing a plague that requires us to reassess and reform some of our cultural and traditional values.

Efforts to prevent HIV have focused on three areas: a reduction in the number of sexual partners, monogamy and fidelity in personal relations, and the use of condoms. It is estimated that approximately 60 to 80 per cent of African women who have contracted HIV have had sexual relations only with their husbands. Because African tradition compares a childless couple to a tree without roots, it is no wonder that couples infected with HIV continue to have children, many of whom are also HIV-positive. These parents subsequently leave behind many children when they die.

It is true that dependence, poverty, and sociocultural factors enable the transmission of HIV to women. But not every African woman is faced with all these problems simultaneously. I believe that every woman must carefully assess her situation so that she can prepare a personal action plan to contribute to the fight against HIV.

As to economic dependence, many women have declared that they cannot change their situations because they depend entirely on their husbands. With this in mind, we must prepare our children, our daughters, our younger sisters, and our nieces to become self-sufficient.

In the face of the HIV epidemic, we women must take charge of our lives. There is an adage that says that one must choose the lesser of two evils. In other words, it is better to stand up for one's right to life than to die young or, through no fault of one's own, to become a widow, sometimes ill, destitute, rejected, and ostracized by society. In the presence of HIV, women must cease living from moment to moment. We must ask questions that address our families' future and seek a model for collective action in which women can unite to change male sexual behaviour. We must refuse to be a link in the HIV chain of infection and be ever vigilant, because the virus can strike at any moment.

It is our duty to keep alive the memory of all the women who have died or who will die because of this century's plague. We must ensure that women who have been broken and humiliated in a silence dictated by tradition have their voices heard. Let our voices be heard in harmony with theirs as we create a future where HIV no longer has the power to silence us.

14   Dawning Awareness

Letitia Laniyonu, Adeola Peters, and Coyin Oke

Letitia Laniyonu, Adeola Peters, and Coyin Oke are
Yoruba women from the Ibadan area of Nigeria.

interviewed by George Orick

George Orick is a writer and editor for many American
newspapers and magazines. For thirteen years he was
a writer, producer, and news editor for several ABC
network news shows in New York, including "The ABC
Evening News" and "20/20." Orick lives in France.

A number of Yoruba women from Nigeria were asked to
share their insights and opinions about HIV and its prevention. The women, who spoke quite candidly, generally
expressed the view that men's attitudes and behaviour are
and will continue to be a major threat to the health of women
and children in the age of HIV. The attitudes and opinions
expressed by the three women presented here are fairly rep-
resentative of all the groups interviewed.

Letitia Laniyonu

Posters put up in public places say that HIV is a killer disease. It is something that you can come in contact with by
being promiscuous. Apart from that, I don't know what HIV
really is. Some people say it's a virus. Some people say it's something else. From what I have heard on the radio and read in
the papers, it looks as if each sex can pass it on. They say you
can't get it unless you are in contact with somebody who

already has it. I don't know if women can give it to men because we are really not well informed about this disease.

Now, in my own rural area, I don't really see people getting HIV, because we don't have any of these modern opportunities. We don't really have any nightlife. Most of us are farmers. After going to the farm, you come back home. I believe that we haven't got a recorded case of AIDS because our men don't go running after strange women. It is acceptable that men have many wives or mistresses. Most of the men have many women in their own houses. They don't have to go out. The women know one another. If any of them had a disease, the others would know immediately.

But what can we do now that our daughters and our sons are going into the city? What about our youngsters who now see this polygamous life as not so good? They want to show that they are monogamous, but in the end they might make a slip or two, and that slip might cost them their lives. What can we do about it? Information about what HIV is, and how to prevent it, is the first thing we should teach our young people.

I am sixty-four years old and I have twelve living children. My eldest, who was born in 1953, is now happily married with three children. My youngest is fourteen years old. I talk to my children freely about sex, and perhaps that has made me lucky. When the girls began their puberty, I told them about what troubles they could get into through sex.

Not many women will talk openly with their kids about these sorts of things. But I am a trained nurse, so perhaps that gives me an edge over other women. I'm retired, but I still work with women in my rural area. That's how I found out that there's a need for us to talk to other women about giving their children sex education. Not just because of HIV or other diseases, but because most of them get pregnant when they don't want to, or when they are too young. So that's how I started talking to them about sex education. Then when we saw these posters about HIV, we women started talking to the children about the disease too, although we have never seen anybody who has been infected with the virus.

I personally think that prevention is better than cure. The prevention is educating these people about what they are letting themselves into by going around with different men and women. I tell them, especially the boys, that they can wear condoms, which are readily available from our health clinics. We have village health committees, and we are given condoms for family planning, but we still tell the boys to use them to protect themselves from getting HIV. So perhaps if all of us do our own little bits in our own little corners, we can wipe out this epidemic.

Many people here believe that men are made in such a way that they have to be with many women. I think that what we are generally saying is that men have decided to have sex many more times than women. Women haven't changed men yet because they think that this is what men are supposed to do; it's embedded in custom. I don't think men need so many women. Most men don't go out to these women because they really love them. They just do it out of habit. I truly believe that women have the power to change men and tell them to be more mature.

Among my sons and their wives, I can see that they have agreed that they don't want to catch anything—from gonorrhea to HIV. I can see the men agreeing, because now that it is on television, they are scared. I see them sitting down with their wives, holding on to one woman, and trying to get as much sexual satisfaction as possible from this one woman.

The men or young people who will not listen are the ones we are afraid for. As we have read and seen on the television, this thing spreads so quickly that it's alarming. Supposing a man gets infected and he has four wives. That means his four wives are infected, and through them a few kids may be infected also.

Let's say only one person within the family has the disease. All other members of the family will be caring for that one. The care, the money, the time—that's a big problem to families like us, who are just making ends meet. You have to buy a lot of drugs while knowing that this is a wasteful exercise. If it was pneumonia or something else, you'd say, "Okay, if I spend so much money buying drugs, this person will be cured." But we have been told that there is nothing to cure HIV. So while you are spending money and time looking after that person, you are saying, "Oh, I'm just wasting my time. When will he die? When will I be free from all this?" Meanwhile, you cannot kill him, you cannot abandon him. So this is a great problem.

You have to pay to be well. We don't have any free services, no health insurance. So I don't know what the government will be able to do, because right now, they're spending all the money we have for education. We don't even have the resources. If HIV becomes a national burden, it will just be too bad. Many people will just die.

Let's face it, if a crisis arrives, we cannot just abandon those who get HIV. We will have to find a way to care for them, and we must keep praying that one day the researchers will find a solution to it. This is why I have stressed the point that education for prevention is the best thing we can do right now.

Adeola Peters

I am thirty-eight years old and I've been married for eleven years. My husband works with the civil service. I completed a higher diploma in secretarial and administrative services, and

I work as a conference coordinator. I have three living children, all girls, who are eleven, ten, and six years old. As of

today, I am the only wife of my husband.

I'm not a Muslim; I'm a Christian. But as you know, when your husband is in a comfortable position, anything can happen. I don't pretend that he wouldn't have girlfriends. I wouldn't say I ever saw him with one, but I assume that he could have one. It is the vogue. Men feel that they should have fun, and there are certain places they don't want to take their wives. If a friend is organizing a disco, in African countries, men don't take their wives, because they feel that respectable women should not be there. So they have people they go out with. If a man has a girlfriend, before you know it, she might be pregnant. Then the African tradition comes in, because once you have a child for someone, automatically you cannot do without the person. So the child can bring you together. That's why I'm saying, as of today, I'm the only one. I don't know about tomorrow.

I don't believe that because he has a girlfriend I should have a boyfriend. What am I looking for? My husband takes good care of me. I am not lacking. If it's attention, he gives me attention. But I think there are things that can push a woman out. Women are not wood; we need attention.

As for my knowledge, from what I read in the papers and from a film on HIV, when a woman has sex with a man, she can get the virus. It takes two people to contract it. Kissing is not part of it. It has to be physical, you know, sexual. And I know they said that once you have it, you don't just die immediately. It gradually becomes more serious, and it may take a couple of years before you die. You start to feel that you have a headache or you have a body ache; then you find that the illness doesn't go away, that it leads to compound illness. I don't know if it's true.

I haven't seen anybody survive or heard of anybody who ever survived it. I saw a film of a Ghanaian girl who didn't survive it. At the last minute, she was very, very lean; like a skeleton.

They say it originates from the United States. In Nigeria we never had anything like that, but they say it's because people travel to America and to European countries. We have many of our people going there to work, some going there for holidays. We can't do anything about that; it's modernization.

I always warn my husband, "Look, if you are going to one of your parties, remember to carry condoms. You know if you die, I don't eat good. The children will suffer. So please remember to carry condoms. Let me die naturally, not from something you have gone out and brought back to me."

He buys condoms. He also used them with me when I was not ready to be pregnant and I was not used to all these tablets they say are precautionary measures. He doesn't really like using condoms, but that is what I want. He will say he doesn't feel comfortable with it, but I don't feel comfortable taking pills. What if I take a pill and die today? He is realistic, so he agreed with me.

Now that HIV has arrived, I think the majority of the men are very cautious. Even those who were carefree before are thinking twice. We have had a reported case of a man who died here from HIV. And since African men are very fearful, I think this will teach them a lesson. We don't have to preach to them. I tell my husband I'm just helping. I'm just reminding him and I'm putting the responsibility on him: "Don't go and get drunk and say you forgot to use it. Don't come into this house and carry nonsense into the house." So he knows and he will be cautious.

Our men today pretend a lot. They will tell you they don't have two wives in the house, but then they go out having girlfriends. HIV will change the culture. It will make them understand that they have to stay with the wife they have known for a long time, and not risk everyone's life. Nobody wants to be looking death in its face like this.

I used to tell my husband, "The day you come into this house and bring a woman and say, 'Listen Adeola, I have decided that this woman is now my wife,' then I know that everything is finished, because I won't have peace of mind." It's not that I'm possessive; I just don't like problems. You start all that nonsense about who did this and who did that. And he knows it's not just a matter of boasting. I value my peace of mind more than anything. I cannot compromise this. I'll leave and divorce him if I find that my life is endangered.

So I should wait until he brings HIV in and gives it to me before I speak? No, I value my life and my children's more than that. If I say "Don't do this" and he continues, and I have a feeling that what he's doing endangers us, I'll leave. We came together because we listened to each other and respected each other's point of view. Let him put himself into my shoes. I mean, if he were me, would he take it?

When the fire is coming into the house, you don't want to sit down until you are burned before you start screaming.

Coyin Oke

I'm thirty-five years old and I've been married for nine years. My husband is thirty-five. He is an engineer and lecturer at the Kwara State School of Technology. He is a Christian, but not committed. I am a committed Christian and the only wife.

We have two girls; one is six and a half, and the other is five years old. When they are older, I will tell them about many diseases, including the one that is spoken of now called HIV.

I will tell them to be careful; before they get involved with any man, they should know that he is serious about them. Since I have put them in the will of the Lord now, I don't think they will rush at anything, especially men.

I've spoken to some people about AIDS. They told me it is an American name that is short for acquired immune deficiency syndrome. But people here don't see it as such. They see A-I-D-S as American Idea of Discouraging Sex.

Some Nigerians I have spoken to believe that there are so many diseases—even worse diseases—that people here must worry about. So this disease that Americans have brought, this thing that kills, well, they would die anyhow. No matter how long they live, they will die of something, so they don't believe there is AIDS.

I believe that this disease exists. In our church they came to show us something about how it affected somebody in Ghana, so I believe that there is a new disease, and I would pray not to have it. But you see, our men, especially the Yorubas, don't cooperate. There's nothing much a woman can do about that. When you tell them to use a condom, they begin to feel maybe it's you. They want to know why you should choose for them. A Yoruba woman doesn't dare to even advise her husband about sex or to use a condom, if she wants them to stay together.

Some men even believe that when they talk with their friends, their wives cannot contribute; that is the place they put women. But things are changing now. Things are changing now. I'm changing also. Before, I wouldn't have left my husband in Ilorin at Kwara State and come to take a job here. Now women are getting to be independent, even the Yorubas. If I see that he's associating a lot with women, and it can affect me, I will just get a divorce. Oh yes, I'm saying I would. Or I would just leave him and say, "Well, I can't have any affair with you; since I had this number of children, I think I'm satisfied."

144

I know how much he earns, and I know how much he's committed to us. He gives us the monthly allowance, takes care of the children, and pays their school fees. If I see that he is lacking in his commitment, I would definitely know that he's spending his money on other things. And no Nigerian woman will do any fun for free. It's for money. When I feel it's getting like that, I'll talk to him. I've caught him once. I paid him a surprise visit and I caught him with a lady. He was surprised and angry that I came without notifying him.

I believe that God can protect me against HIV. He can protect my husband. If God loves me so much, and if He sees that I don't do anything against his wishes, He could, because of the love He has for me, protect my husband. I keep to myself. It's only my husband I'm not sure of. So that's the problem. How can I safeguard myself against that? He wouldn't wear a condom. If I refuse him, that would create a problem. Then he's going to stop coming here, and the children will start asking questions. My parents would also get involved. How would I raise my children? He would divorce me. Maybe I should just start talking to him and saying, "If you want to have an affair, think of us and make sure you wear a condom."

15 Positive Dialogues

Margaret Mwangola

*Margaret Mwangola founded the Kenya Water
for Health Organization (KWAHO).*

Rose Mulama

*Rose Mulama is the KWAHO programme
manager for the Lake Victoria region.*

interviewed by George Orick

*George Orick is a writer and editor for many Ameri-
can newspapers and magazines. For thirteen years he
was a writer, producer, and news editor for several ABC
network shows in New York, including "The ABC
Evening News" and "20/20." Orick lives in France.*

Margaret Mwangola is a liberator. She has liberated approximately 1 million women from the time-consuming, mind-
numbing work of carrying water daily from rivers and ponds
to their villages. Given clean water—the prerequisite of good
health—and released to redirect their time and energy, these
village women have created an ecosystem of development.
Schools rise, gardens thrive, waterborne diseases diminish,
longevity increases, and profits from new small enterprises
organized by the women are invested in community projects.
Says Margaret Mwangola, "The African woman who does not
go to the river gives birth to a new woman."

This interview took place during a two-week visit to
KWAHO villages in western and southern Kenya. For three
days of that tour, Margaret was accompanied by Rose Mulama.
Rose, a sociologist and single woman, brought a different

145

generational perspective to the discussion the two women shared about HIV. They spoke of a growing awareness of the epidemic among the women of KWAHO villages, citing in particular the village of Kakamega, near the Kenya-Uganda border.

Rose: HIV is a reality now. It's in our midst. As we see our own relatives dying, we have begun to accept that we must take preventive action and also provide care for those of us living with this disease.

Statistically, it's difficult for me to say where it's more prevalent. It's very difficult to determine whether it's a town or a rural problem. Within our African setting, when people are infected, they normally go back to their rural communities to die. So even if they got infected in the urban areas, the impression is that there are more cases in the rural areas. This is why, over a year ago, the women in the village of Kakamega decided to organize themselves to do something about HIV. They decided to come together to talk about how HIV is spread and what they could do to prevent it by working together and making their husbands aware that if people were more faithful to each other and could stick to one partner, then we would be able to reduce this epidemic.

It is a good thing that polygamy is dying because of the economic situation. Men cannot afford to have two or three wives anymore. One wife is more than enough.

Margaret: In your generation, my darling. Someone died last week in my church, and no one knew he was a polygamist. We cannot deal with the present and not deal with the past.

Rose: It's so difficult to actually guarantee that a man is not still going to go out with other women. This is our problem.

Margaret: He will go. That's the problem.

Rose: The issue is not polygamy anymore. It's the issue of people accepting that HIV comes about by not having some self-control. If people can appreciate that aspect, then I think it will help.

Margaret: I agree, but in Africa it will never happen because of the upbringing of our men. They're led to believe they are kings for the women. So we must also deal with the root problems.

I come from the coast, where polygamy is not strong, but some of my people are Muslims. My sisters-in-law think I'm very lucky because my husband has never thought of it. Maybe I'm too much of a handful and will not allow polygamy to take place in my house. That doesn't stop me from feeling for my sisters-in-law who are in this situation. If you are lucky, you can control your husband, but you control him within your house, within your bedroom. It is the society that controls the man, and therefore we have this conflict.

Rose: In the past, maybe some women were content with the fact that they had no control over their men. He owned the house and he owned the bedroom. The woman just didn't want the headache of chasing him around to find out what he was up to. Then HIV came in, and now people are nervous. It's not an issue of control anymore; it's an issue of when he returns, you may be a victim of something you have not actually participated in. This is what is making people like the women in Kakamega start to address what can be done about it.

Margaret: I couldn't agree with you more. If I may speak for the married women, they are now more worried than the single women. If you are unlucky, you may have a stubborn husband who is ready to die from HIV anyway, so he will go with anybody he wants. Yet as a married woman, you are trying to be very careful, trying not to have another partner in your married life. Because of your husband's attitude, though, you can die. It's a very frightening experience.

And in our marriages, you do not necessarily stay with your husband every day. The husband can be in Mombasa, the wife can be in Kakamega or Machekos. And chances are that the man has several affairs. So the woman is in a very difficult position.

I would recommend this: if any education about HIV is to be done, it must be addressed to men first. We women want to care for our families, our brothers and sisters, and the people around us, but our lives can be cut short by someone who is careless—someone who claims to get drunk and not know what he's done afterward. And you, the wife, are in a very helpless situation.

Even as much as women in the Northern countries claim to be controlling their men, there is also this arrangement of having mistresses. So I do not think the women in the developed world are as powerful as they want us to believe. There is something we share: unless a husband is completely faithful to you, I think we are all singing the same tune. It doesn't matter what age—the husband can bring it home.

If my husband wanted to be a polygamist today, I don't have one traditional power to stop him from doing so. In modern Kenya, I could stop it because I want him for myself, for my children, and for our home. At the same time, he could keep me and still keep mistresses—one in Mombasa, one in Kisuma, and another in Nairobi. In that case, I'd be very happy if he officially became a polygamist. At least then I would know who the other woman is.

Traditions that could be useful in this area should be looked into. At my age, I'm trapped in between. I cannot be the modern woman. I must address both worlds. When I go home, my aunt who never went to school still goes to the river a mile away to fetch water. I must walk with her, and I must carry the heavier calabash of water while she carries the lighter one. We return home talking. Instead of being an executive officer in Nairobi, I'm now a real African woman, serving my aunt. The international community expects me to behave like an executive. An executive of what? When I go back home, I must be my traditional self.

Rose: When we work with these communities and their water problems, it brings them together as a group with a common goal. One of the issues we address is reducing the burdens the women face in terms of water collection: the time they spend, the distance travelled, and the risks involved in drawing water. Once they are relieved of these problems, they have time to sit down and look at other serious problems that are affecting them and see what they can do about them as a group.

Margaret: The major emphasis of our programme has been on maintaining water sanitation between the tap and the mouth: the containers we collect water in, the boiling of water at home, the use of sand filtration, or what can we do to prevent waterborne diseases within the village. Through this process, we bring more awareness about HIV. I don't want it to supersede all other health issues, but I agree that it's a very important thing.

Rose: AIDS takes time before it really germinates; we all may look healthy, but we don't even know if we have the virus.

We do not have drastic numbers of deaths, one after the other, but the women can see that it is happening elsewhere. They want to take precautions.

That was a very big step for them as a community. They're trying, in spite of not being fully informed about the disease. You can hear some of them saying, "It may be coming out of use of dirty water, use of latrines, and so forth," which is not true. In spite of that, they're still making efforts to educate one another. I think that is the major first step. From a village point of view, they have really made progress.

Margaret: Extension workers have also supported the villagers with health education material. They are urging doctors and health-care workers to hold forums and discussions and are calling for seminars and workshops to go into more detail regarding how the community can protect itself from HIV. Not all organizations in Kenya are involved in these activities; there are specific ones such as the Red Cross, Family Planning Association, and health-sector nongovernmental organizations that are mandated by the Ministry of Health to do this. We in the KWAHO office, for example, can draw upon them only to come and discuss the disease in the evenings and show films, but we do not carry out the HIV prevention programme as such. I've seen that the Ministry of Health seminars include men. So it isn't only the women who break the news about HIV in the villages. We hope that this approach has improved the dialogues within homes and families.

With more people becoming educated and aware now, and more exposure taking place among families, women are travelling to the cities to attend seminars and conferences. We find positive dialogues, even when some husbands and wives do not have effective communication at home. HIV has brought about discussion. Everybody's afraid for their lives. Now it's very fashionable to talk about the disease, what is going on, and how people are dying. However, very few of us really understand what's going on.

In most African countries, sensitive issues related to sexuality and childbearing have never been the subject of easy discussion in any home. This is a very private cultural matter. It embarrasses everybody. Family planning was impossible to introduce in Kenya because, many years ago, there were tribes that wouldn't talk about controlling births. So you have to face cultural difficulties.

Rose, you are in the age group of my daughter. In traditional Africa, I cannot discuss issues related to sexuality with my daughter. My husband's sister or my sister discussed that with her. But in modern Kenya, I can do it. My sisters will not come to Nairobi to talk to my children. I can't find the time to go to my sisters' houses and discuss these things with their children. And my aunt is too old and too busy to come to the city.

So we parents of today are left with no option but to be friendly with our children, to discuss their personal secrets with them, and to try to help them. I have teenage sons. Each time they want to enjoy themselves I tell them, "You have to be careful because it is no longer safe nowadays." Traditionally, I would never do that; I would have no business telling my sons to be careful. But if they go out and become infected with HIV or my daughter does, who is the loser? Is it not me? So I have said to hell with the traditions. I must tell my children.

Rose: I support that very strongly. People cannot handle HIV as a secret thing anymore.

Margaret: The women talk. I do not imagine that they have the factual knowledge to carry out serious discussions of this subject, because many of them don't understand Kiswahili or English. But the information process, as disorganized as it may be, cannot be dismissed altogether. I think the word is spreading: "There is this disease. Look after your daughters. Look after your sons. Be careful of your husband if he persistently comes home late. Maybe it's good to talk to him."

This is now going to bring in the use of condoms. Eventually, the old myth about men not getting their satisfaction with condoms will be overturned. Lives will be saved—if condoms do save lives—because satisfaction and sexuality are just at the back of your brain. I want to believe what doctors and nurses are telling people—that the chances of preventing HIV are greater if condoms are used. But you don't just come into a village and begin to discuss issues related to sexuality. HIV will not give women the mandate to control their husbands. Maybe insights and ideas on how to approach the subject quietly with their husbands would help.

Rose: I think influencing the husbands is one thing, but controlling them is another. Sharing the problem with them and sensitizing them to its seriousness and its effect on us and the family are more important than trying to seize control of their habits. They're human beings; they have a capacity to listen. They are also being affected.

Margaret: Then there is the issue of the people who have someone sick at home. This is very hard: the moment you announce that Margaret Mwangola has become infected with HIV, because of the way it has been perceived, people run away. The person living with HIV becomes a severely isolated, medically feared person, whom nobody wants to be near. Then the agony the family goes through, let alone the sick person, is unbearable. Something ought to be done to bring positive education to everyone.

153

Rose: The major problem is how we can help those who are living with the disease. We all know how difficult it is to provide care and counselling, especially in a rural setting where there are other illnesses like diarrhoea and dysentery. I would appeal for some kind of assistance to give that kind of support and to try to create more awareness of prevention in rural communities, particularly for those who are not yet affected and for the younger generation.

Margaret: I can tell you quite frankly, I'm so afraid of this disease. I don't stay with my husband, and I don't have the ability to check his movements; so, like the village women, I am afraid too. And because I am dreading it, it must affect my relationship with my partner.

I can assure you that AIDS information, the way it has been mishandled, has created more separations and divorces than ever before. People are full of distrust. They're full of fear, and they're not enjoying themselves because they're waiting to be told that they are positive. It used to be syphilis; now we've got a killer disease. And who is going to be responsible for these broken marriages? It's bad enough, without the AIDS component, that a lot of husbands and wives are not talking.

How do you expect widows to manage their lives without one or two boyfriends? How do you expect women who are frustrated in their marriages to manage their sexuality without a boyfriend somewhere? How do you expect a man who is a widower, or a man who can't get along with his wife, or a man whose wife has a medical problem not to have a partner?

If I was told that my sister had AIDS, my immediate reaction would be, "Oh, poor Mercy, what will she do?" All the neighbours would run away from her. Her husband would also run away from her, and maybe her children would leave. Who would help her? If I touched her, would I also get it?

Why all these negative feelings? For goodness' sake, whoever discovered HIV, please discover a way to put across hope for the future.

Until now, the whole approach on this issue has been completely wrong. Instead of making us all aware and careful, people have been instilled with fear. People are afraid of one another, afraid of those living with HIV, and afraid of getting the disease from their husbands and wives. If fear were dispelled, it would lead to positive education and prevention, which would be much more effective.

Rose: I don't think the issue of where HIV came from is very important. If the white man or the European continent is so disturbed about the deaths caused in Africa by this epidemic, what are they doing about it?

Margaret: It's no use sitting in New York, Paris, or Copenhagen and assuming that anybody who is a community leader, or in an executive position, is knowledgeable about AIDS. Maybe there should be a major campaign of basic preventives, basic information kits that can be given out in churches, schools, youth clubs, the scout movement, nongovernmental organizations such as KWAHO, and government ministries. A package that tells you how you can deal with it, whom you should go to first, and how you can prevent spreading it.

Rose: It's the hopelessness we all feel that makes people just say, "Okay, let me tackle it sort of individually." Then, in the final analysis, we realize that this is a very slow and defeatist approach, because we do not live in isolation. If you're married, you cannot guarantee 100 per cent that your partner won't cheat on you. So it is helplessness and hopelessness that make people shrink back and not get involved. This has created more ignorance among us.

How do we help one another to accept that the disease is here; that it is happening because of a, b, c, or d? We need to share and accept this as the world's problem and march together to find a solution to it. If it means more research on how to cure the disease, if it means support in terms of strengthening the preventive measures, then this is what we are calling for.

We are asking, "What's the outlook?" The United Nations Development Programme, for example, is concerned about this problem. What kind of support can it come up with? How do we support those who are already living with HIV? How can we address ourselves to the present before we think of the future, especially when everyone is fearing that the entire human race is going to be extinct, or that by the year so-and-so half the population or the younger generation will be wiped out?

Margaret: Even if we can gather millions and billions for AIDS programmes, unless they are implemented with the full participation of the recipients, they will be a waste of time. They can keep their millions.

In Kenya, we have taken positive steps to curb the spread of the virus. The Ministry of Health is spending millions of shillings on education every week. Everybody's being encouraged to help educate people, create awareness, and become volunteers.

I must see to it that KWAHO and community leaders within KWAHO play a substantial role in community awareness, community health education, and HIV prevention. Through our unified action, it may not take long before

we reach a point where we can triumph over this disease. There will be no wiping out of the world.

16 Self-Esteem Is Essential

Patricia Burke

> Dr. Patricia Burke was programme director of the Family
> Centre of the University Hospital of the West Indies, a
> nonprofit organization that provides care for per-
> sons living with HIV and AIDS and their families.
> As a member of the National AIDS Committee of
> Jamaica, Burke is responsible for the development
> of national HIV and AIDS policy guidelines.

interviewed by Berl Francis

> Berl Francis is a Jamaican communications specialist
> with more than twenty-five years' experience in
> the fields of public relations and journalism.

My first contact with HIV in Jamaica was totally unexpected.
For several months during 1987, my colleagues and I had been
investigating the cause of a three-year-old child's persistent
cough; her enlarged liver, spleen, and lymph nodes; and her
general failure to thrive. We conducted a battery of tests, but
the source of her illness remained a mystery until I attended
a lecture by Dr. Celia Christie, a Jamaican who had recently
returned from studying infectious diseases in the United States.
Then I realized that the child had AIDS. That was the first
case of paediatric AIDS in Jamaica; within a few months, we
identified four more.

HIV is viewed by most Jamaicans not as a virus that causes
chronic illness with remissions and exacerbations but as an
acute plague, a scourge, a moral blight. The society regards
itself as highly religious and morally upright. Thus HIV is
viewed as a disease of homosexuals and commercial sex workers, as they were the first people to be publicly associated with

the disease. The conclusion many people draw is that people who contract the virus deserve their lot. Our homophobic society is quick to point out that in the Bible, the punishment for sodomy is death.

Although government studies indicate that the majority of Jamaicans place more credence on advice from physicians than from any other health-care professionals, to date, there has been little concerted effort from that quarter to educate the public. The majority of doctors are male, and I suspect that their reluctance to speak out is based on a fear of being labelled homosexual.

In this atmosphere of ignorance and prejudice, rejection of those living with HIV is almost automatic. Stigmatization is the last thing that HIV-infected persons and those diagnosed with AIDS either want or need. The fear of discovery, stigmatization, and censure has sent many infected and affected people underground to protect themselves. They would rather be dead than rejected.

People diagnosed as being HIV-positive react like anyone faced with grief and loss. They show the classic responses of denial, anger, bargaining, depression, and acceptance. But in light of society's strong censure, they also show tremendous paranoia. Because this is a small country, their first and foremost concern is that no one should know.

Are Intensive Information Programmes Enough?

For the sake of those who are infected and also for the good of our entire society, a much more intensive information programme should be launched immediately. We must educate the public about the reality of the disease and the necessity of treating people living with HIV and AIDS with compassion and understanding. Current information programmes are helpful, but HIV cannot be controlled through mass media alone. With the media, one is simply transmitting a message. Information is disseminated but unless attitudes and concepts are changed, behaviour will not change. The basic concepts affecting self-esteem, sexuality, and disease prevention must be addressed before behaviour change can occur.

Our country desperately needs a national education programme that focuses on teenagers and younger children. Classes that teach about human sexuality in the context of awareness and responsibility, provide information on sexually transmitted infections, and destroy myths that encourage unsafe practices must be developed.

Targeting this younger age group is especially important in Jamaica, because early sexual activity is a distinct aspect of the social and cultural pattern. Nearly 25 per cent of all births on the island are to girls ranging in age from ten to nineteen. It is expected that by age eighteen, the average young woman will already have given birth to two children. Currently, young adults between the ages of twenty and thirty-nine constitute the most highly HIV-infected age segment of society. Given the incubation period of HIV, it is clear that many became infected as teenagers.

Attitudes and behaviours within a society are so deep-rooted that they are extremely difficult to change. Counselling sessions that address activities that put people at risk of contracting HIV and self-esteem-building programmes are needed for both men and women of all ages and all socioeconomic groups. For example, among middle- and upper-class Jamaican women, there are many whose sense of self and social status are tied to marriage. If a woman, regardless of her economic class, can be encouraged not to barter sexual favours for money and status, then she may feel more secure in telling a man to wear a condom.

In our society, men's self-esteem is closely linked to their sexual prowess and to the number of women that they can support financially. Men are also taught that sexual experience and the ability to control women are valuable male characteristics. Mothers and fathers alike encourage that sort of behaviour as their sons grow into manhood. The more financially successful a man is, the greater his sense of entitlement. If men can be encouraged to value sexual responsibility and restraint rather than excess, we will have gone a long way toward reducing the risk.

We at the Family Centre have watched self-esteem-building approaches work with family members of teenagers living with HIV. When the centre first opened, we recognized the need to involve these adolescents in various activities. Unfortunately, many young girls believe that their only means of escape from poverty is the commercial sex industry. Girls who come to the Family Centre are being shown that there are other options through unstructured, ongoing interaction with the programme staff. Gradually the girls begin to adopt new attitudes toward themselves; as a result, new behaviours evolve. When interacting with males, the girls now tend to be more assertive and self-confident.

People attending the centre are drawn exclusively from poor economic groups, which are hardest hit by HIV. Illiteracy and the absence of marketable skills heighten their vulnerability. But there are also a number of other factors at work that contribute to the problem.

Male response to economic hardship may well be a contributing factor to the instability of so many relationships. For most men, unemployment and underemployment are the norm, and their wages often provide only the basics. In the rural areas, many choose to become migrant workers. They work on farms in the United States and Canada or in the cane fields in their own or neighbouring countries. They tend to establish relationships with women wherever they go. As a result of this migratory lifestyle, serial relationships often become a way of life for low-income Jamaican men and women.

Other factors are involved, however. One of the most important is socialization. Girls are taught from an early age to develop strategies for survival, which usually revolve around their ability to work, to be caretakers, to market sex, and to bear children. The latter is very important, because men place a high value on proven virility. As a result, women who do not bear children risk being labelled "mules" and being abandoned. They are not seriously considered for marriage. At the same time, girls are taught that it is extremely important to have a male partner, that men are dominant, and that a woman is not free to do what she wants but must "take telling" from her man. So girls are socialized to be economically and socially dependent on men.

Boys are not taught to be caregivers, and they are not taught to be fathers. Too often they are encouraged to believe that their sexuality and promiscuous sexual behaviour are a measure of their manhood. Boys are not taught survival skills the way girls are. In the absence of this training, they depend heavily on the women in their lives, but they are unhappy about it. They have internalized the ideology of male dominance, but they resent their dependence on women.

Unemployed men are economically dependent on women. Their feelings of depression and inferiority in this situation are manifested in repeated abuse of the women in their lives. This abuse can be both physical and psychological. He may beat or rape her; he may constrain her freedom; and he may develop relationships with a number of other women.

It is significant that in Jamaica heterosexual men have the highest rates of HIV infection. This situation has serious implications for women who engage in unprotected sex. Currently, the number of women infected with HIV is rapidly increasing.

Although pregnant women are not routinely tested, those whose behaviour or clinical history suggests possible exposure to HIV are usually tested when they visit a prenatal clinic. If a woman is found to be HIV-positive, counsellors will inform her of the risk to her health and the risk that her child will be born with the virus. She is allowed, but not coerced, to make a decision about terminating the pregnancy if it is in the very early stages.

Jamaican women who live in poverty tend to be malnourished. In a family where food is limited, the male head of the household traditionally receives the lion's share; the children get the next-largest share, and the mother takes what is left. The effect of such poor nourishment on infected women, who are responsible for the care and nurturing of their families, is that they tend to die faster than men. This may also be exacerbated by the fact that infected women often put their own health needs behind those of their family and may not seek medical help until the disease is more advanced.

What of Tomorrow?

Historically, Jamaican women have been unable to depend on their mates for their families' financial needs. Thus, female heads of households are a dominant fact of life in Caribbean societies. As a result of the HIV epidemic, trends strongly indicate an increase in deaths among women who are heads of households. They will leave behind infected as well as uninfected children. An increasingly heavy burden will be placed on relatives and friends who will be called on to care for surviving children. We have tried to tackle this serious problem by initiating a fostering programme, but our resources are limited. We are experiencing difficulty in raising funds to feed parentless children and adults who are without sources of support.

I look ten years down the line, and frankly, I am terribly concerned. My worst fear is that Jamaica's already fragile family structure will unravel. We will have more parentless children, an increasing number of homeless, an increase in commercial sex work born of the desperate need to survive, and the consequential and continued spread of the virus.

Many of the infected people I work with can repeat verbatim the information about how the virus is transmitted, yet they continue to have unprotected sex. They fear the consequences of disclosing their HIV status, or at the point of actual sexual contact, they become intimidated by the mechanics of safe sex. Unless one has practiced putting on a condom, doing so for the first time at the point of arousal can be difficult and frustrating. Many women have never even touched a condom. And despite the efforts of our health-care professionals to educate them, many men do not know how to use condoms either.

If nothing is done to change the attitudes and behaviours that perpetuate HIV, we will have a nation populated with impoverished young and old people. We have already seen evidence of this in parts of Africa. I do not want to give the impression that HIV and AIDS are problems only of the poor. The "haves" in our society are also stricken. For the more affluent, the consequences are likely to be as devastating. Those who can afford available medication are spending more than

U.S. $25,000 a year. These treatments may prolong their lives, but they will eventually die, and the money that might have gone to educate their children will have been consumed by medication.

HIV seems to be spreading faster in the poorer nations of the world than in the rich, but there is only one world. Events and developments that take place in any one part inevitably affect the whole. Countries that have more resources should help stem the disease's spread in poorer nations by contributing financial support and expertise.

Countries like Jamaica must recognize that HIV is not to be trifled with. The disease must be treated as a national concern, not a government, health-sector problem. In Uganda, HIV is no longer viewed as strictly a health problem. The government has taken an aggressive stance toward the disease, and all government ministries are involved. Here in Jamaica, the private sector is already getting involved, albeit to a limited extent. Our National AIDS Committee, which has a heavy representation of private-sector interests, is responsible for advising the government on HIV-related issues, but the programme has few resources.

People are creating programmes to fight HIV, but efforts are fragmented, and I fear that there is much duplication of effort and a subsequent waste of limited financial resources. We need to delegate responsibilities to various agencies acting under the direction of a central government agency, which would also coordinate the procurement of funding assistance.

In spite of the gravity of the situation, there are positive aspects to this challenge. The public health sector is doing a valiant job in the face of daunting odds. We have an excellent blood-bank system, and no infections through the use of blood or blood products have been reported since 1985.

If the collective will is mobilized and we pull together, we can eliminate some of the conditions that enable HIV to flourish in our country. The old saying "United we stand, divided we fall" has taken on a very special meaning for me as Jamaica confronts HIV.

17 We Must Be a Caring Society, Not a Scared Society

Prateep Ungsongtham Hata

> *Prateep Ungsongtham Hata was born and raised in Klong Toey, where she established a school in the hope that education could transform the lives of children and lead the way to development. She won the Magsaysay Award in 1978 for her work and used the proceeds to establish the Duang Prateep Foundation (DPF), which has become a major force for slum development in Thailand. The foundation's HIV and AIDS project is a community-based programme run by local volunteers. This essay was written with the assistance of Julia V. Bindman, a former DPF volunteer, and Jenny Godley, a former DPF staff member.*

By the end of the 1980s, the myth that HIV was not a Thai disease was shattered by alarming figures showing the spread of HIV throughout our population. Today, although estimates of incidence vary, two points are clear: the country is in crisis, and heterosexual contact is the major mode of HIV transmission.

Silence and denial characterized the government's initial response, prompted by fear of the disease's impact on tourism and foreign investments and by an official reluctance to acknowledge the presence of a booming commercial sex industry. To date, preventive measures have been minimal and largely ineffective. Few programmes have been developed for either HIV-positive people or those who have been diagnosed with AIDS.

The spread of HIV in Thailand is primarily a result of the powerful but illegal commercial sex industry. Contrary to popular belief abroad, and foreign press statements notwithstanding, the overwhelming majority of clients are Thai men, not foreign tourists. When it became socially unacceptable for Thai men to have multiple wives, the habit of frequenting brothels became an accepted practice. A Thai man who does not visit commercial sex workers after the age of fifteen is not considered a man. By the time they reach the age of nineteen, more than 90 per cent of Thai men frequently interact with commercial sex workers. Visiting brothels is a socially accepted activity, usually preceded by an all-male evening of dining and drinking. This custom crosses all social and economic boundaries.

A tacit, fundamental national belief exists that men and women have different sexualities. Men are seen as needing sex and a variety of sexual partners. Women are expected to remain virgins until marriage and are assumed not to have sexual needs or to enjoy sex. Sex is rarely discussed between men and women. Although women often joke about men's "bad habits" among themselves, most accept this behaviour and consider it preferable to the potential rivalry of an additional wife. In the context of the Thai male's demand for an industry that ensures the availability of sex outside of traditional relationships with women, HIV is clearly a cultural issue.

There are both economic and cultural reasons for the overwhelming numbers of Thai women who are now sex workers. The national development policies of the past thirty years have led to rapid, but geographically uneven, economic growth. The resulting decline of agriculture and the disintegration of rural society have caused economic hardship and cultural changes. Migration rates have soared as young people move to urban areas in search of jobs that will enable them to send money home to their parents.

Thai Buddhist culture stresses the importance of loyalty to parents. Sons can show filial gratitude by becoming monks, but no similar spiritual solution exists for daughters. Tradition demands that they provide for the material needs of their parents and families. Young rural women, newly arrived in the cities, have little access to well-paid employment. Commercial sex work is by far the most lucrative job that a woman with a low-level education can find.

As rural impoverishment intensifies and the demand for consumer goods among villagers grows, the commercial sex industry will continue to expand, and with it the spread of HIV. Thus the epidemic in Thailand is also a development issue. Today, many nongovernmental organizations (NGOs) throughout Thailand are focusing on HIV, attempting to fill the gaps in public services by providing education, counselling, and support systems. The Duang Prateep Foundation (DPF) was one of the first to address the issue. At the foundation, we recognize that although HIV and AIDS are international problems, the issues surrounding HIV transmission and medical treatment vary across local and national boundaries. It is in this light that we wish to share the experience of our community-based development organization as we work to fight HIV in Klong Toey, Bangkok's largest squatter community.

Klong Toey

Bangkok has a population of approximately 9 million, representing more than a tenth of Thailand's total population. It is estimated that 20 per cent of Bangkok residents live in illegal squatter settlements. Klong Toey, which is located next to the harbour on swampland belonging to the Port Authority of Thailand, has existed for more than forty years. Approximately 60,000 of Bangkok's low-paid workers have built homes here that are accessed by a network of wooden boardwalks traversing swampland and rubbish heaps. The people live mainly in extended family groups organized along the lines of a traditional village.

Klong Toey is divided into eighteen subcommunities, each with an elected council that receives limited recognition from public authorities. The residents are always vulnerable to eviction. Overcrowding strains such basic services as drainage and refuse collection and threatens the safe-water supply.

Both within and outside the community, the residents are almost universally regarded as second-class citizens with no hope of improving their circumstances. Persuading them to abandon this view of themselves is essential to any form of community action or education.

The easy availability of drugs around the port and a desire to escape the harsh realities of Klong Toey life have contributed to a high incidence of drug use. DPF first became aware of the presence of HIV in Klong Toey in May 1988, when intravenous drug users attending the foundation's Freedom from Drug Abuse Programme were tested. Thirty-six per cent were found to be HIV-positive.

Initially we thought that HIV in Klong Toey would be too large a problem for an NGO to manage. However, the lack of government response to HIV and our unique position in the community, coupled with a sense of responsibility to those around us, led us to establish the HIV project. The philosophy behind our project reflects not only our commitment to community-based action but also a realization that Thailand's medical system is ill equipped to cope with the morbidity and mortality associated with this epidemic.

Any campaign to mitigate the effects of HIV must focus on preventing transmission and on promoting social acceptance of people living with HIV. Moreover, since habitual male use of commercial sex services puts every member of society at risk of infection, we regard HIV as a social rather than a medical problem. The project's aims are to teach people how to protect themselves and their families from infection; to promote understanding, not fear, of people living with HIV; and to provide practical assistance that will enable such people to live in a supportive community.

After ensuring that our own staff was fully informed about HIV, we held street parades with educational messages displayed on floats and banners and sponsored prevention slogan competitions in local schools. Most of our educational activities have been aimed at teaching intravenous drug users, their families, and commercial sex workers how to protect themselves and how to pass this information on to others.

We started with intravenous drug users and focused on prevention by offering counselling and general information about HIV, AIDS, safe sex, and needle sterilization. We also provided health checks, blood tests, free condoms, and bleach to decontaminate needles and syringes. An educational campaign aimed at commercial sex workers in the community was launched in September 1990. As with the drug users, most of the commercial sex workers were known to us through our networks in the community, and we visited them where they worked.

We secured the cooperation of brothel owners and local police in encouraging women to attend our information seminars and recruited two female sex workers to receive further training as peer educators. Despite DPF's urging that men who refuse to use condoms be turned away, many of the women cannot afford to do so. Nor can those who know that they are infected afford to stop working. Studies in Chiang Mai and Ratchaburi provinces indicate that brothel policies of "no condom, no sex" can be successful if they have police support and if every brothel in the province adheres to them.

Strict Thai social rules concerning status and respect place a commercial sex worker at the bottom of the social scale, leaving her powerless to insist on condom use. Meanwhile, the male customers, who refuse to use condoms and sometimes even offer to pay more for unprotected sex, have been exempt from criticism. We thus decided to make male customers the focus of our next campaign, starting with the young men who provide cheap motorcycle taxi service around the area. Seventy-three per cent of the 489 questioned said that they visited commercial sex workers regularly. Eighty-seven drivers attended the first training session in December 1990 and were taught how to protect themselves from infection and how to pass on safe-sex messages to their customers. They were also issued brightly coloured vests bearing our anti-HIV logo to raise public awareness.

Education for the entire community, especially through peer groups, is the focus of our current campaign. Because Klong Toey residents often feel marginalized and disconnected from the rest of society, they are inclined to believe that information "from above" or from outside the community is not applicable to them. The peer-group approach is therefore more successful, because it helps people relate the information to themselves and their lives.

We actively seek volunteers from the community. We began with fifteen *mae bahn* (housewives), who attended information sessions and shared what they learned with friends and neighbours. We also send mobile teaching units door-to-door to ensure that information is disseminated throughout the community, not just to those who choose to obtain it.

Currently, most people living with HIV are still asymptomatic, and some are reluctant to acknowledge their illness. We have expanded our work to assist them in coping with life with HIV. People practicing high-risk behaviours and identified by community contacts receive home visits from volunteers and are offered counselling and support.

Indifference to HIV, despite local and national education programmes, is still the prevailing attitude. Even those who are fully informed about the disease, its transmission, and the eventual symptoms do not, on the whole, perceive themselves to be at risk and have not modified their behaviour. Among men, peer pressure to be "manly" and reluctance to change habits are still stronger influences on behaviour than fear of HIV. The widespread belief that the king's daughter (currently involved in HIV research) or foreign doctors will soon find a cure also diminishes fear. It is possible that people will take HIV more seriously once they see many members of the community falling ill and dying. Today, more immediate threats such as eviction, fire, and unemployment, and more common illnesses such as hepatitis, take priority.

The biggest challenge we face in our work is winning and maintaining the trust of intravenous drug users and commercial sex workers. Their experiences with other agencies tend to make them suspicious of everyone except their peers. When our need for data in planning the project led us to accept outside assistance, we experienced comparable problems and attitudes. The aims of academic researchers did not always coincide with ours, and their inappropriate and intrusive questioning damaged our relationship with the Klong Toey population. We are working hard to restore trust within the community, and we now treat data collection more cautiously.

Being singled out for questioning on serious and personal issues is a disturbing experience for any Thai, putting him or her in an inferior or defensive position. The Thai concept of *kreng jai*, an awareness of social hierarchy and one's place in it, combined with the desire to please or placate one's superiors, means that answers are often tailored to please the interviewer rather than express the interviewee's true thoughts. Because we do not wish to subject members of the community to a demeaning experience or damage our relations with them, our information is gathered through informal interviews, stories, and impressions collected by project workers. The foundation's efforts will continue to focus on education. We will also continue to develop appropriate teaching materials. These are the key to our efforts, although some of the existing materials are not as effective as they could be. Our aim is to educate everyone in the community to protect themselves and to accept people living with HIV. We want to encourage and support families in the community who are taking care of their loved ones, and we plan to open a community support center to provide education and counselling for families of people living with HIV.

At the Duang Prateep Foundation, we believe that our resources are best used in educational campaigns. Other agencies, with appropriate expertise and funding, must assume the responsibility for providing financial aid and medical assistance to the ever-increasing number of us who are infected with HIV.

What of Tomorrow?

Within the Klong Toey community, we expect an increasing incidence of people with AIDS in the next few years, as intravenous drug users, whose immune systems are already weakened, begin to display symptoms. In the near future, more people, including commercial sex workers and their clients, will also need medical attention. We foresee that housewives and the babies they bear will soon be severely affected by the virus.

We have no way of knowing when large numbers of mothers and infants will begin to show symptoms, nor to what extent our prevention programmes may have protected them.

Thailand may mirror the experiences of some African countries, with equal numbers of men and women contracting the virus, a high rate of perinatal infection, and many children left parentless.

The economic implications of the epidemic in Thailand are appalling. The cost in terms of lost productivity will be massive as the virus takes its toll on Thais of working age. Perhaps the worst effect will be when investors begin to lose confidence in Thailand and its future. Foreign investment, tourism, and demand for Thai labour abroad may decline if Thailand is seen to have a large HIV-positive population. The impact of an economic recession on Klong Toey would be enormous, because poor areas are invariably the first to suffer.

The financial strain on the health-care system will increase yearly. By the year 2000, more than 500,000 Thais may have died of HIV-related illnesses, and many more will be ill. The health-care system is obviously ill equipped to handle an epidemic of this scale. The generally poor level of health and sanitation throughout the country, especially in the slum areas, leads us to believe that the life expectancy of people living with HIV in Thailand will be low.

Family and community ties have always been strong in Thailand, and this is highly evident in Klong Toey. The economic hardship and social discrimination that people living with HIV and their families may face will severely strain these ties. In Klong Toey, care for those diagnosed with AIDS will, in most cases, be provided by the family, which may face a seriously lowered standard of living. The wage-earning capacity of the ill person and his or her family custodian will be lost, with severe consequences for families already struggling to survive.

Women, as traditional caregivers, will be the most heavily burdened. Support will be needed for the parentless children who are infected and for their healthy siblings as well. In many instances, grandparents or other relatives will raise them, but others will become street children unless alternative caregivers can be found.

The Thai tradition of the extended family may be threatened by the epidemic, separating people spiritually and socially and turning a caring society into a scared society. To avoid the breakdown of these ties, building community acceptance and understanding is important. Buddhism teaches tolerance of others and compassion for the sick. It will be important for the *Sangha* (our highly respected Buddhist monkhood) to take an active part in promoting a supportive attitude toward people who are HIV-positive.

Eighteen of the most prominent NGOs have formed a coalition known as the Thai NGO Coalition Against AIDS. Many of the members of this coalition believe that commercial sex work must be legalized in order to slow the spread of HIV. Absolute enforcement of the use of condoms will be possible only if brothels are under strict government control.

The key to halting the spread of HIV in Thailand does not lie in discouraging men from visiting brothels. Behavioural change on such a large scale involves changing the fundamental nature of relationships between men and women, which would simply take too long. In the short term, the epidemic must be stopped by encouraging men to use condoms. All sexually active women must be empowered to insist that men wear condoms. Sex education, including information on safe sex practices, must be offered in the schools and through public education campaigns. New employment opportunities must be made available to Thai women as alternatives to commercial sex work. The roots of the epidemic lie in Thailand's socioeconomic structure, and it is there that solutions must be found.

18   Moving from Fear to Hope

Ian Campbell

Ian Campbell, the medical adviser for the Salvation Army, develops health programmes internationally. From 1983 to 1990, he worked at Chikankata Hospital in Zambia, where he was involved with all areas of HIV prevention, care, and counselling.

During a visit to Norway, I was asked to address a group of high-school staff and students about HIV. At the beginning of the discussion, the students chose *fear, confusion,* and *death* as words to describe their feelings about HIV. At the end of the session, the words they chose were *inclusion, community, choice, challenge,* and *hope.*

This new choice of words reflects a transition in thinking and emotional investment. It also reveals the capacity of a small group of people to concentrate realistically on the global impact of HIV and to relate it to various aspects of development. These people are no longer observers; they have become active participants in problem solving. They are incorporating suffering and loss while gathering resources to deal with the impact of this disease. The group members were not only discussing hope for other communities but also demonstrating real hope for themselves and using their own previously unrecognized internal resources.

Hope lies within each of us in the exploration of these resources. Some communities in southern Africa are already exploring their resources, and their experiences have much

176

to offer those in the First World who are in similar circumstances. Theirs is a framework of hope that requires an honest grasp of the relational and spiritual issues we face when dealing with HIV.

Some words speak in special ways. They have influence. I will focus on *inclusion, community, normalization,* and *hope.* All are conceptual yet practical, abstract yet concrete. They are words that arise from four years of experience in HIV programme development in southern Zambia and, more recently, in other parts of the world.

The Influence of Inclusion

Privatization is usually practiced under the guise of respect for personal rights. Yet the shame, fear, stigma, and confusion of HIV will not end with strident, moralistic imperatives about human rights. However, in every crisis there comes a time of helplessness and a need for burden sharing instead of burden bearing. This is true for HIV. Constructive, respectful, and confidential information sharing about HIV is needed. Most importantly, there is much we can learn from the experiences of people who are living with HIV.

Care programmes cannot operate effectively in a vacuum. If we care for individuals in their home environments, the family becomes interested in problem solving and, in turn, the community develops a concrete interest in HIV prevention.

Integrated HIV management is necessary to promote a coordinated approach to care, prevention, and control. It is a multidisciplinary technique that is committed to both task and process, but not in a technical manner. A fusion of problem-solving approaches that apply to different categories of human need is required. Obviously, clinical care is necessary for HIV-related illnesses, but counselling is also needed for someone living with HIV who needs support and information when he or she is ready to approach family members. In turn, the family needs to know how to respond to this situation, how to face the future, and how to turn a problem into an opportunity for themselves and their community.

Relationship values, spiritual motives, and integration of life should all be preserved, provided there is a means of incorporating and resolving the problems that arise as a result of HIV. This will not happen without an applied approach to information sharing that is agreed upon by all, helpful to all, and concerned with problem identification and problem solving. This is often where counselling, including community counselling, comes in. The inclusiveness of counselling is demonstrated in the capacity of a community to meet, examine, and make choices about its collective future.

These choices ultimately focus on behaviour change; this change resides with each person, involves the family, is affected by the community, and is subsequently transferred to the nation. Counselling is the primary tool for behaviour change, community development, pastoral care, and education. Southern African communities are usually willing and able to deal with the issue of behaviour change. This is because a respectful dialogue is the priority. Behaviour change for the individual, the family, and the community occurs by inclusion, not by intrusion. It occurs through recognition of mutual accountability. When the responsibility for behaviour change is accepted and acted upon by the community, room for an external facilitator can be created.

Trust enables the participation of an external facilitator to be effective. It is an essential part of the counselling process. Yet gaining the trust of an entire community can take considerable time to achieve. More often than not, trust is established through the compassionate demonstration of care for someone who is ill.

Yet the spread of inclusiveness—generating a wave of energy for change, survival, and even growth in relational values—cannot rely entirely upon the energy of the individual. Inclusion requires political leadership and support from the highest levels of government. The power of example is great, and truthful politicians are needed—politicians who respect and value honest relationships with communities, institutions, and nongovernmental organizations.

Inclusion means confidential sharing, which is an apparent paradox. It means preservation and growth in relationships rather than disruption. Inclusion means developing a network of support through respectful burden sharing rather than intensifying personal stress through isolated burden bearing. It means the inclusion of people related by family groups as well as those who are bound together by mutually shared objectives.

In turn, nongovernmental agencies that are active at the community level should continue to express their needs to those in the international arena that possess the financial resources and influence desperately required to continue their work. International organizations often operate without the involvement of those working in the field or those who are living with HIV, but these are the very people who have the greatest capacity to solve problems because of their experiences.

Inclusion also implies inner security and a readiness to accept the diversity of human life. Inclusion recognizes the capacity for spiritual life in others and recognizes the importance of maintaining a quality of life that accepts and transcends the difficulties of living with HIV. At a time of crisis and pain, the spirit of inclusion is the most basic building block of successful programme development. Inclusion recognizes the fact that the best begins now with oneself and with others.

The pastoral-care presence is part of the spirit of inclusion. For the majority of people living in developing countries, the recognition of spiritual life is not a conscious process. Spirituality exists from birth for the individual and is incorporated into everyday life.

The Influence of Community

HIV affects individual relationships as well as those of a larger community. It is a false assumption that all groups in Africa automatically function well as communities. They do not. Each person within a group has his or her own agenda, and each group has its collective agenda. Communication is needed to progress from a group consciousness into a community awareness that solves problems in the interest of all its members. Thus, the capacity for community consensus, specifically the capacity to agree on approaches for a collective future, is another major building block for programme development that Africa can demonstrate to the rest of the world.

This community awareness is also of major importance when developing and implementing HIV counselling. Counselling interventions at the community level depend on community centredness and participation for their success in the same way that one-on-one counselling depends on client centredness. Most importantly, effective counselling can be created only with the participation of members of the community that it is supposed to serve.

Many programmes focusing on HIV-related issues in southern Africa began as a result of research interest rather than the desire to establish care programmes. Great skill is required for programmes that are attempting to encourage community awareness of research objectives, because the community is not interested in research objectives. It is concerned about who the beneficiary will be and whether it should participate in these programmes.

A community understands its limitations; thus the facilitator team should also declare its limitations unequivocally. Often the facilitator team, whether focused on research, home care, or education for HIV prevention, is more concerned with the implementation of the project. These efforts can result in failure if the team is inflexible in this regard. This failure is preventable if the team recognizes that it is in partnership with the community and, as such, can afford to reveal its weaknesses and learn from the people it is working with.

This is one of the strengths of the Chikankata Hospital HIV care and prevention team in Zambia. Its example is being shared in HIV management training seminars. Health-care teams train for five days at the hospital and then conduct field visits. Most participants recognized the need for a transition in attitude from being a provider team to being a group that gives what it can, but receives what it should from the group with which it works. This is an example of the concepts of mutual interdependence and inclusion in community.

Our task is to encourage community development by defining the community and facilitating its success when it is working in its own interest. Community development approaches to HIV prevention are less likely to destroy hope and sabotage community initiative than many past attempts at primary health-care implementation. Communities throughout the world need to shift power from the health-care system and authority structures to themselves. This is true empowerment, because the capacity to act is acknowledged, confidence is asserted, and participation has begun.

What is actually happening with communities in southern Africa is happening in other areas of the world, with people who understand the challenge involved in helping a potential community become a functioning community. Africa can teach us this by example. To many in the First World, this is unexplored territory, because it is assumed that hope for community was lost long ago. This is far from the truth. Community affirms choice and incorporates challenge. It is the most effective tool we have to eliminate confusion and fear.

The Influence of Normalization

If we are honest, we can acknowledge that we deny and avoid problems when they have a significant impact on our lives. This is also true for nations as they try to deal with HIV. A syndrome of rejection and denial can be discerned in people's reactions to HIV at the national planning level.

Nations in southern Africa have accepted malaria and other diseases as reality. HIV is very different from these other diseases, but it needs to be incorporated into everyday life, just as they are. This does not mean that we accept HIV or that we are losing hope for its control. It means that we are being honest.

Tactical support mechanisms such as condoms, vaccines, treatment, and needle-exchange programmes will never control HIV, although they will prevent its transmission. They need to be placed into a broad strategy for prevention, and this requires realistic, honest thinking.

The fact that HIV affects relationships and is integrated into value systems and behaviour requires that it be normalized. But it usually is not. Tactical maneuvers become detouring panaceas. This happens because HIV is not acknowledged

Ian Campbell

honestly, particularly in the First World. There is widespread
superficial recognition of the presence of HIV, but little else.
Normalization happens more easily in the context of the cultural depth and diversity found in southern Africa, where
people discuss not only the quantity of the problem but also
the quality of the response needed.

At this point, the presumption seems to be that vaccines
or treatments will not prevent or cure HIV. If Zambia, for
example, has experienced difficulty in achieving 40 per cent
vaccination coverage for measles after spending millions of
dollars, then clearly a vaccine will not solve Zambia's HIV
problem. Neither will a vaccine or treatment solve the United
States' or Britain's HIV problem, even though it is commonly
assumed that they will. Such assumptions should be avoided
at all costs. We must honestly recognize, and not just verbal-
ize, the fact that HIV is part of our lives.

Many people working in development claim to be aware
of their involvement in the international context of health-
related community development. However, this internationalism is rarely felt and reflected in programme designs that
incorporate both a caring spirit and skills in strategy development. HIV has disrupted this complacency by demanding
internationalism at its best. In this sense, there is no other
option for the future. Development of positive relational
alternatives and subsequent choice making about sexual
lifestyle, survival, and growth strategies is an absolute necessity for HIV prevention and control.

Yet it is apparent that people, communities, and countries
do not realize that they have a choice. The inevitability of HIV
need not be depressing, provided it is recognized and integrated with an increasing awareness of a capacity for choice
making about the specific issues of relationships and sexual
expression. In one sense, there is no choice, but in a truer

sense, HIV can enhance liberation by clarifying the choices that are actually available for people. The extent to which some African countries and communities are normalizing HIV is a strength and a challenge. This is what needs to be communicated to the First World.

Honest normalization contains a capacity for respectful choice, for incorporation of suffering, and for problem solving through development of the concepts of inclusion and community. Normalization contains a commitment to inner security that is based on awareness of the value of the work of others, and training programmes should be shaped by this awareness. Africa's ability to normalize HIV has implications for training programmes throughout the world, because they too should contain a commitment to power sharing, inclusion, community, and survival; to quality rather than quantity; and to comprehensiveness of vision rather than restriction to personal agendas or narrow issues. The challenge of HIV is unavoidable, yet we can choose the methods we employ to deal with it.

Those with health training and other forms of expertise are also needed as part of the team of problem solvers. This includes people who are living with HIV. All of us are decision makers, and as such, we are responsible for discerning these choices.

The Influence of Hope

Hope is the basic building block of life. It is measurable through the establishment of programmes that work by promoting strategies for behaviour change that can be implemented realistically. Through action, energy is generated for the unseen future.

Faith in the unseen is another form of hope. Sometimes acceptance of the difficulty of life in southern Africa is assumed to be fatalism. It is not. This acceptance can take the form of faith in a future characterized by the sharing of human and spiritual resources, by inclusion in community, by honesty and integrity. Hope is the courage to believe that life is a mystery. Hope is the knowledge that we are going somewhere.

Moving from paralysis to action is a move from fear to hope. Yet mysteriously, concrete action that speaks to people, particularly those who are living with HIV, begins with a belief that there is hope for a solution. HIV was not sent to us for a specific reason, but we can use it to help us move toward that solution.

19   I Can See a Light at the End of the Tunnel

Noerine Kaleeba

> *Noerine Kaleeba is the director of The AIDS Support Organization (TASO), the first organized community response to the HIV epidemic in Uganda. TASO now provides over 6,000 people living with HIV or AIDS and their families with counselling, information, medical and nursing care, and material assistance.*

My personal involvement with HIV began on a June day in 1986 when the virus entered my front door. One year later, the disease had taken my husband, leaving my four daughters and me to struggle with the social ills of this epidemic. Since founding The AIDS Support Organization (TASO) after the death of my husband, I have been exposed to the numerous questions that HIV and AIDS force our world to confront. I have also experienced the joy and satisfaction of watching the Ugandan people in particular, and Africans in general, move away from paralytic shock to organized, positive response to the disease.

My first encounter with a person living with AIDS was very brief and promptly dismissed. Today the experience is vivid in my mind. I was at Mulago Hospital demonstrating the practical techniques for transferring a paraplegic from a bed to a wheelchair. A young man who could not have been more than thirty years old gave permission for my students to learn from him. His medical notes indicated that he had paraplegia due to immunosuppression syndrome, but I was unfamiliar with the diagnosis. I later spoke with the ward nurse regarding the scheduling of the demonstration. She warned me, saying, "I wouldn't touch him if I were you. He has AIDS. We don't touch him, we only show his mother what to do." I cancelled the class and arranged for another patient volunteer without ever giving the young man an explanation. I did not think of him again until my husband was diagnosed with AIDS. To this day, I wonder what happened to him. I wonder if he and his mother had anyone to support them and help carry their burden. I suppose I will never know.

TASO began as an organization that provided counselling and support facilities for people with HIV and preventive counselling for families and communities. Our aim was to impress upon people in the community, especially at the grassroots level, that a person who is HIV-positive or is diagnosed with AIDS is not dangerous. At the time that TASO became active, HIV was becoming a reality throughout the world. People were beginning to react and to initiate responses to the epidemic. Many of these initiatives were focused on prevention, which we at TASO believe is a good approach to an incurable disease.

Unfortunately, the public health messages at the time were very negative, associating HIV and AIDS with death and low morals. Nothing positive was being offered to those who had already been diagnosed with HIV, and these messages only served to further stigmatize and torment them. This is why TASO adopted the slogan "Living Positively with AIDS." We called on everyone in our society to be compassionate and supportive toward those of us who are living with HIV, and to join us in a collective fight against the disease.

Today TASO is a nongovernmental organization (NGO) that offers counselling services, outpatient clinical care, and home care for people with HIV and AIDS. We also offer awareness and sensitization programmes for a cross section of the community, from medical personnel and political leaders to village community workers.

Over the last four years, we have intensified our efforts to educate people to the fact that HIV is an infection and has brought a new dimension to our lives. Increasingly, people are having personal experiences with HIV and AIDS through affected family members or friends. And they are beginning to realize that they cannot catch HIV by sitting next to someone who has it. In areas where we started TASO community programmes, villagers are beginning to accept that HIV is in their midst.

In Uganda, when someone is ill, all the villagers come to express their sympathy. With HIV, people stopped doing this because of fear and because they did not wish to offend by saying the wrong thing. The villagers now ask, "How do I visit my neighbour and begin to discuss HIV?" There is also a feeling similar to the one the late Philly Bongoley Lutaaya expressed in his song: "Today it's me, tomorrow it's someone else." People are saying, "If I am not kind, if I do not sympathize and get involved with my neighbour, what will happen to me when my turn comes?" So increasingly, people living with HIV and AIDS are being supported and cared for; many more are coming out and saying, "I have HIV."

In TASO, there is a group of about thirty people living with AIDS who are willing to discuss their problems openly on the radio and television. Whenever I speak publicly, two or three of them accompany me, because people will not relate to what you are saying until they have actually seen a person who is living with the disease. In the beginning, people with HIV and AIDS were seen as dying, but we emphasize life rather than death. It is the quality rather than the quantity of life that is important.

In many countries, the level of HIV infection is high. We cannot ignore people who are HIV infected anymore, the way we did when we were first exposed to this virus. The Ugandan government's approach to this disease has had to change as well. For example, in 1986 and 1987, there were discussions about mandatory testing and isolation of people who were HIV-positive. Eventually that talk stopped, because the reality of our situation is worse than was previously thought. If everyemployee at a major institution like the Central Bank was tested, and three-quarters of them were infected, would the bank be closed? It became quite clear that strategies such as mandatory testing would be ineffective and expensive and would provide little in the form of alternatives or improvements.

Only a comprehensive prevention programme of care, support, and counselling will work in our society. This is even more evident if one examines the nature of HIV. People do not know that they are HIV-positive until long after they have become infected. I believe that communities are fed up with HIV prevention messages that do not offer concrete followup. When a villager receives counselling and support, the community is being sensitized to the fact that a person who has contracted HIV is not guilty of any offense. HIV is a disease that thrives on secrecy, and the only way we can fight it is to do so in public, enlisting as many members of our communities as possible.

The combined strategy we are employing in Uganda may be useful for other countries as well. First we started with awareness. There are still areas of our country where people are unaware of many aspects of the virus. They have heard the HIV warnings on the radio and the slogans such as "Love carefully." But the awareness they need begins with question-and-answer sessions that encourage them to understand what HIV and AIDS are about. After we have accomplished that, then we offer counselling, testing, care, and support. A combination of all these approaches is what is needed.

This strategy works. Villages surrounding Kampala and as far away as Kumi, in the eastern region, are recognizing the need for a collective effort. Recently, a delegation of elders from Kumi asked us to start a community programme for them. Almost every week we receive teams from other countries—for example, Botswana and Zambia—who are trying to understand what we are doing. These are some of the many areas that TASO has become involved in as the organization has grown and adapted to the needs of our communities. One of the advantages that NGOs have, unlike the Uganda AIDS Commission, is that we can plan as we go along. We are not afraid of making mistakes. If we had planned everything in advance, TASO would never have been started.

HIV is caught only in specific ways. The fact that TASO teams go into the homes of people who are living with HIV and come out intact sensitizes the community to concentrate on the most important mode of HIV transmission: sexual contact. We offer counselling about behavioural change, especially for those of us who are infected, but we also keep in mind that this change does not happen overnight. We know that this counselling is producing positive outcomes when we look at the group of people living with HIV and AIDS in TASO. Even if they do not specifically tell me that they have changed their behaviour, the fact that they have spoken publicly on radio and television about their HIV infection is proof of change. They have, in effect, warned anyone who is not HIV-positive not to have sex with them. People are making important and responsible decisions about their lives.

We are also seeing a dramatic reduction in pregnancies among young infected women. This is because our counselling is targeted toward helping people make conscious decisions about their lives. In Africa, it is a real behavioural change for a young woman in her mid-twenties to decide not to have a child.

In my experience, the people we support at TASO have generally not indulged in risky behaviour. What they have done is find partners who are also HIV-positive. They do not have multiple sex partners. A person with HIV has the right to have sex, but it is important to impress upon people that they are responsible for not passing their infection on to someone else. Some of the questions we address are: When you are with your husband, what do you do? What do you do when you do not have a partner?

Our counselling emphasizes the rights and responsibilities of people who are living with HIV. Simply stated: If I have a right to live, then I also have the responsibility to let others live. For people living with HIV, the first goal is to treat opportunistic infections and then try to boost their immunity. But above all we reassure them that they are not dying and that they can live with HIV and AIDS. After just the first counselling session, they feel much better.

It is important that those who are infected understand that people care for them. If they feel that they are being scorned and are considered dangerous, their sense of responsibility toward others erodes, and they become angry. This is why we encourage a more caring attitude in public.

There are indications that behaviour is also beginning to change among those who are not infected, though this information is mostly self-reported. People are saying, "I know HIV is out there, and I am being careful." In 1990, we opened up the first voluntary and anonymous HIV testing and counselling centre in sub-Saharan Africa. We were unsure whether anyone would use the facility, but today we are overwhelmed. The turnout is very high, especially among young people.

I was exposed to HIV because my husband was infected. My first test was negative, but I was encouraged to be tested again in six months. I have not yet gathered the courage to take a second test. Whether the results of our HIV tests are positive or negative, we must conduct ourselves so that we avoid becoming infected or spreading infection. For people to have the fortitude to walk through the door and get tested and counselled, they must have made a decision to change their lives. One thing you do know is that once you walk out that door after being tested, you will never have unprotected sex again.

The responsibility of saving lives is an individual one. The best TASO can do as an organization is to provide as much information and counselling as possible through various channels, including discussion, radio, and television. Now we are providing information through the mouths of people living with HIV. But it is up to the individual; you are the only person who can save yourself. Sex is an activity that takes place behind closed doors.

For many of us, changing behaviour is a gradual process. Yes, we are hearing about behaviour change among men. But polygamy is a part of our society, and it will take intensive programmes to help men adapt. There are many traditional practices that are in direct conflict with the messages we are giving. We must educate people to understand that what they lose by ceasing a traditional practice is less devastating than what they may lose by contracting HIV. This process will take time.

Changing behaviour is not very difficult; keeping it changed is. We should motivate people rather than threaten them. We must constantly strive to develop positive messages. As people get tired of one message, throw in something new, something different, to keep up their morale.

When addressing women, I ask them to reward men with love rather than threatening them. Besides, how many women in our culture can afford to be that assertive? Women like myself, who have an income, can pick and choose. But then there are those like my sister in the village, who live at the other end of the spectrum. I have discussed HIV with my sister and given her condoms. She has never been able to show them to her husband because she is afraid of being thrown out of the home. In our culture, once a woman is married, she must have sex with her husband whenever he demands it. She cannot negotiate safer sex without risking her very existence.

I am also very concerned about the vulnerability of my daughters and other young women. Older men are pursuing sexual relations with girls and young women more than ever before, as a means of preventing HIV infection. I worry about these young girls, who are increasingly becoming victims of rape and sexual abuse and who cannot protect themselves from HIV and other sexually transmitted infections (STIs) in these circumstances.

I have become involved in empowering women to defend themselves against HIV. Women are beginning to demand new laws that protect their rights against abusive husbands and traditional practices that relegate them to an inferior social status. But passing laws is not enough. Women must be taught how to use these laws to defend themselves. Family members, elders, and the community must also support these laws.

There are many ways to organize different members of our society. Official programmes, such as educating a gathering of 100 people at the local elected councils, have their role, but by themselves they do not create awareness. What is more useful is training one person from their midst and sending that person back with some incentive to spread the relevant information. This is cheaper than organizing rallies and paying the allowances of Ministry of Health personnel. These educators would be willing to work for 2,000 to 3,000 shillings per month, compared with the monthly government salary of 12,000 shillings.

In every African village there is a storyteller, a person to whom the villagers can relate. Train that person, supply him or her with a uniform or some other form of identity, and you will see a change. Groups of people who are already employed in community programmes or local committees can be trained and given some incentive to continue the work. Eventually this type of programme could be employed throughout the country.

When I think of the impact that HIV is going to have on the coming generations, I become very emotional. I truly do not have a vision of what will happen. In Uganda, death and dying are issues that affect children directly. There are many children who are parentless. This is the result of our political situation as well as the epidemic. Though we lost our home when my husband died, my own children have not suffered so much materially, but emotionally they are devastated. They not only lost a father to HIV but also carry the stigma of the circumstances of his death. My daughters are not like other children who are parentless as a result of HIV; the others do not have a mother who goes around talking about HIV every day!

Most parentless children lose both parents to HIV within a very short time. They cannot go to school or get enough to eat. They are going to be emotionally and socially different from other children of their age groups. Recently eighteen children came to TASO from Mbale (in the eastern region), where they had been living in foster care. They had already lost so much time from their lives. All the plans that World Vision, TASO, and other organizations are making to support them are being implemented too slowly. These children are growing older, and they cannot switch off their growth until we finish planning. One of the early discussions we have with people living with HIV is about what will happen to their children. We impress upon them that they have a fatal illness and must begin planning for the future to ensure their children's survival.

At TASO, we recently began a pilot project to create income-generating activities for our clients living with HIV. This programme involves relatives who sign contracts obligating them to be responsible for our clients' interests after death. We are conducting this on a small scale, because these activities can be complicated; many people use the money to meet their immediate needs rather than saving it for the future. We must investigate more efficient types of income generation to assist surviving relatives who are burdened with unplanned HIV-related responsibilities.

In Africa, the HIV epidemic appears insurmountable because it is compounded by so many other issues. The North-South imbalance is highlighted by HIV. Today our hospitals still lack medicine for preventable diseases. We know that one of the cofactors in HIV transmission is STIs, but we still do not have a comprehensive STI control programme in Uganda. Another means of exposure to HIV is the blood supply. Our blood bank is still inadequately screened, but this too could be accomplished with adequate funding.

Despite all the problems we face, when I look at the future of HIV in Uganda through the eyes of someone who works with people who are living with HIV and AIDS, I see a ray of light at the end of the tunnel. The initial fear of rejection that kept so many of us in hiding, and therefore made it possible to infect others, is now disappearing. We no longer have to fight this virus in isolation. Each of us can join together to ensure that our hopes for a world without HIV become a reality.

20   There Are Lessons to Be Learned

Theresa J. Kaijage

Theresa J. Kaijage is the founder of WAMATA, a Tanzanian advocacy and counselling group for people infected with HIV.

HIV has taught African communities a few lessons, the most important one being that they must raise a unified voice and stand up for themselves, because no one else will do it for them. Communities have become aware of the need to supplement government efforts to promote HIV intervention efforts at the grassroots level, and as a result, HIV service organizations have begun to form. Some of these organizations comprise people who are infected with the virus, and others include their families as well.

The AIDS Support Organization (TASO) of Uganda, under the leadership of Noerine Kaleeba, has taken the lead in HIV support in sub-Saharan Africa. Its counselling services provide relief for many infected persons who are living positively with the virus. Similar efforts are emerging in Kenya, Zambia, Zimbabwe, and other countries in the region.

In Tanzania, WAMATA, a Swahili acronym for People's Groups Fighting Against AIDS in Tanzania, brings families together for mutual support, care, and counselling. When WAMATA was founded in June 1989, it was a desperate attempt to intervene in a critical situation. Today, whenever possible, we provide economic support in addition to counselling and social services.

During the last few years, the WAMATA has adapted to the process of engaging in family intervention. First, WAMATA counsellors have learned that it is preferable and more productive to engage both partners in counselling before one of them dies. This helps the partners resolve their anger and various conflicts as it prepares them for the difficult task of preserving the rest of the nuclear and extended family. Facilitating the family's and community's process of coping with a member who has contracted HIV can be a challenge, but it is important to prepare people for the situation.

Because the ideal situation of intervening before one partner dies rarely presents itself, counsellors are usually in the position of helping the surviving partner mourn and prepare for his or her own impending death. They must also address the needs of other family members, because it is often through the surviving spouse or partner that a family first learns of HIV in its midst.

WAMATA members have learned the importance of linking the care of soon-to-be parentless children to the care of an ill parent. Children must be supported during the terminal stages of their parents' illness and prepared for a different life. This gives the biological parents an opportunity to stimulate their children's bonding with parental substitutes, and it encourages mutual trust to develop before both parents die.

The person living with HIV should also be encouraged to develop a positive attitude toward living, even if life may seem difficult. An individual may wish to enter into a legal union with a partner on whom he or she can rely for support when confronting the disease. Family members, legal counsel, and religious institutions may be brought in to execute the couple's decisions. Counselling at this stage may involve exploring available alternatives for preventing HIV transmission to an uninfected partner.

WAMATA has come to appreciate the value of linking preventive services to supportive care and counselling, because it is through the latter that individual contexts of behaviour and behavioural adaptations can be addressed. Mass education is important, but it is not an end in itself. Socially learned behaviours are acquired over a long period of time, and relinquishing them is also a gradual process. This may require various types of assistance, the identification of which usually occurs in counselling. Learning and sustaining new behaviours may also warrant professional support. A relapse in HIV-preventive behaviours is different from a relapse in other chronic problems. With alcoholism, for example, chances for regained sobriety still exist after a relapse, as long as therapy is assured. But a relapse into unsafe sexual activity could lead to infection with HIV, which is incurable. I am always hopeful that people, once they see an example, will be more committed to taking their lives into their own hands and shaping their own destiny.

It is difficult to single out HIV as one problem rather than part of a complex set of problems. Since the arrival of HIV, it has become more apparent that those living in developed countries may benefit from identifying with their counterparts in developing countries. One way to do so would be to join us in our struggle not only against HIV but also against conditions of poverty, which enable the disease to thrive. Greater intergovernmental and interagency collaboration is needed if we are to overcome this epidemic.

Development assistance of today is policy oriented, and some of the policies are laden with postcolonial power imbalances. The issue of partnership between North and South must be addressed if we are to avoid reinforcing the status quo. Neither donors nor recipients of development aid will gain from more of the same.

Currently, development assistance is being rerouted through nongovernmental organizations (NGOs) instead of through governments. One of the stated reasons for this is the avoidance of government bureaucracy. But I believe that the North prefers to fund NGOs because they require less funding. Moreover, although they choose to bypass governments, Northern funding sources demand the same type of bureaucratic structure from grassroots NGOs. The result is that NGOs in developing countries are competing for scant resources, yet a high demand is placed on them in terms of managerial ability, financial accountability, and proposal writing.

In the long run, this situation could lead to funders sending their own staffs to direct programmes in developing countries. Are grassroots NGOs capable of managing themselves? Or will they be funded only if donors send their staffs to oversee operations? In the latter case, a good percentage of donor funds will go toward sustaining their own personnel at much greater cost than hiring local employees. Conceptually, this scenario is fine if the outside staff is sensitive and empowers the organization so that the local staff quickly becomes capable of operating without outside supervision. But usually this is not the case. Once the recipient organization's employees become dependent on an outsider's instructions, they do not develop their own skills or the confidence to make mistakes and learn from them. Whether outside management can create sustainable development remains to be seen.

There are communities in which everybody knows everybody else and shares some form of identity in the network of relationships based on either kinship or good neighbourliness between villages. If we extend this good neighbourliness to the global community, we may find a way to identify with one another and join in our common struggles against HIV and against the conditions of poverty caused by global economic inequalities. Development assistance programmes, if grafted onto such inequalities, will succeed only in reinforcing the status quo, which is the very cause of uneven development at micro and macro levels.

To limit the waste of resources—especially time, which is absorbed by administrative functions—we should all collaborate. For example, at the donor level, there could be a clearinghouse for funding agencies to share funds among NGOs rather than encouraging competition. NGOs and national education and prevention programmes should share tasks and information that link them beyond national borders.

It is difficult to meet the needs of donors and simultaneously justify the needs of recipients when providing services to the client population. For example, there is pressure from all quarters to emphasize the role of survivors, particularly parentless children, rather than caring for the ill. Yet in my community, it is in the interest of survivors to take care of the sick and infirm. The two functions cannot be separated; therefore, we must link the care of the ill with the care of the grieving. The costs incurred in helping a person live positively with the virus is nothing compared with what that person gives back to the family and community for the remainder of his or her life.

HIV knows no boundaries. All people are equal in front of the virus. Those of us who exist on the margins of society are more vulnerable, and when the stigma of HIV is added to the stigma of poverty, we suffer a double disadvantage. However, we must act quickly to take advantage of the epidemic to advocate for change, now that HIV has given us common ground.

Equal partnership and mutual support ought to be the guiding principles in all human relationships. Only full realization of the give-and-take in our interactions will promote recognition of the value of each person's contribution to the global community of nations.

21   Long Live Life!

Herbert Daniel

Herbert Daniel was a political activist, writer, director of the Brazilian Interdisciplinary AIDS Association (ABIA), and president of Groupo Pela VIDDA (Group for the Proper Appreciation, Integration, and Dignity of AIDS Patients). He wrote this essay in November 1990 and died of AIDS in 1993.

In this narrative I am embarking upon, I will talk about the future. This means repeating what has become my basic message during the past two years: I have HIV and I am alive. This statement, in the simple present, is my celebration of the future. This message, usually followed by a joyous cry of "Long live life!" may seem like a paradox if we let ourselves be guided by the mass of fantasies created during the past decade about this disease and epidemic. For me, this time has been an apprenticeship in living and in hope. To be honest, I cannot say that I have discovered that I am going to die or that I have come to have a more intimate relationship with death. These banalities would not get me very far. What I have discovered is my mortality: the meaning of my own fragility, of my transitoriness, and of my impermanence. Mortality is not something to be confronted in the distant future, for I am now face-to-face with my own future.

As we confront HIV worldwide, we must ask what the future will be for each and every one of us. Many doomsayers

This essay is dedicated to my best friend, Sheila, who, like me, is fond of the Beatles and the Rolling Stones and does not give up.

have sounded their trumpets, pronouncing the epidemic a sign of the end of time—as if it were our failure in the face of a virus that seemed to have a moral objective and a teleological orientation. I never believed these pessimists, for I soon realized the ideological content of their analyses. They are the same pessimists who were always rushing to explain humankind as a consequence of a particular failure at a certain moment of the Fall and sought to reduce our quest for the recovery of a Lost Paradise. Labouriously developed over a ten-year period of renewal of taboos and prejudices, the metaphors of HIV served as a good model, typical of the 1980s, for the mystification of the Fall and Salvation.

Since the beginning of the 1980s, I have participated in HIV information programmes. At that time, their main thrust was geared toward people who had not yet been infected, as the number of infected seemed too insignificant to focus on. It seemed that there was little or nothing to say to those who were living with HIV or those who had been diagnosed with AIDS, except that they were about to die.

That is exactly how I felt when I became ill. Even though I considered myself a relatively well informed individual, I immediately translated the diagnosis of pneumocystis pneumonia into death. My doctor acted strangely and was excruciatingly shy about pronouncing the word *AIDS* in front of me. He referred to "another infection," as if he were under the power of an ancient superstition (some say that the name of the devil should not be mentioned, so as not to invite evil). I knew then that I had a disease whose name was not spoken. Even though I knew much more, at that moment of despair, the prevailing thought was the popular formula AIDS = DEATH. Statistics took on reality in my mind. I became a number, and I concluded that I had two more years to live.

This happened two years ago. I knew at that moment that I was dying and that my days were numbered, rigorously and mathematically. In the midst of my fever, of my crisis, of my awe, I saw myself as benumbed, as someone dying much more from the belief that I was going to die because I was HIV-positive than because I was facing a disease that would consume me.

Then I looked deep inside myself and discovered an extraordinary thing: I was alive. Furthermore, I was going through an ordinary experience, namely, that of dying. It is an experience that all of us, with no exception, will go through someday. Yet for most, it is always in the distance. How was it, I asked myself, that I could go through this experience and not communicate it as something deeply original, to be shared by the ones I love? I felt immediately that I was not dying from AIDS, one of the conditions associated with infection by HIV. I was dying from something else with the same name—a very complex social construct also called "AIDS" that led me to accept ostracism, separation, and banishment. I was dying from what I might call social death, the absence of all human rights. What is it that leads us to alienate ourselves so absolutely from our concrete experiences? Yes, I was very ill. But I was suffering more from the effects of an induced image, a metaphor. A word had been spoken, and it was bewitching me.

My initial reaction was a burst of passion. I said: I am living my life! And I insisted: I am not going to let myself be killed by prejudice. If the virus is going to kill me, let it do so after I have exhausted my resources to achieve a balanced coexistence with it.

That is why I am now going to write about the future. I am forty-four years old. I remember myself at the age of twenty-four, full of enthusiasm for the novelties of the world as expressed by the Beatles. At the time, as a participant in the resistance against the military dictatorship in Brazil, I was condemned to death. At the time, I had a very intimate relationship with death. At any moment I could be imprisoned, tortured, and murdered by the agents of repression who had done away with hundreds of my companions. I escaped. But not without having learned something about death. At the time, I gave little thought to a possibility like this one, of writing a narrative about my country's and the world's expectations for the future in the face of a threat as serious as HIV. It happened, life happened. Many faces appear to me from my past, whispering that death is no big deal. The extraordinary thing is that the lives of the dead continue to provide inspiration for the renewal of hope.

Twenty years later, here I am, imagining the future. As in the Beatles' song, I am imagining twenty years from now, "when I'm sixty-four. . . ." It is extremely improbable that I will be here to blow out the candles on that birthday cake. That is what they say. But it does not matter. Here in the present is where life is and has been happening. I do not know whether I will live to be sixty-four. So I am sixty-four today. At this moment.

I will try to build peace. By dismantling the hostile triggers of the mythology of HIV, I will try to ensure the victory of life. Perhaps John Lennon would appreciate my tribute, but I appreciate still more the possibility, in a text like this, of freezing the trajectory of a bullet from yesterday that is unable to silence a voice today, that still keeps whispering to me, "Imagine. . . ."

Brazilian Time

In order to tell my personal story—that of someone living in a country like Brazil—I have to try to unravel a complex tangle. Long before diagnosed cases of AIDS appeared, the HIV epidemic was announced in my country as something we were fated to inherit from the so-called developed countries, especially the United States. The press and the public were awaiting the first outbreak of what was then being heralded as the gay plague or gay curse. The news was broken with some fanfare after the deaths of a number of well-known homosexuals, who by chance had lived in the United States.

I am emphasizing these facts of history in order to draw attention to the process by which a mythology was built up—a process whose very striking characteristics were to determine the entire future evolution of the disease, right up until the present. The elements of that process were:

1. The exoticism of a foreign disease, virtually a fairground curiosity, that attacked primarily a deeply marginalized and stigmatized group that was usually relegated in the national press to the crime or medical pages. HIV would slowly be built up as a disease of other people.

2. The sensationalism that treated those assigned to "risk groups" as victims of catastrophe, but also as if they were paying the price of a fall. The replacement of epidemiology by victimology went still further when people with haemophilia began to be affected on a broad scale and were quickly categorized as innocent victims.

3. The inevitably fatal nature of the disease, which directly and mechanically associated death—a cruel, inglorious death in a hospital—with behaviour patterns that were termed marginal: sex, pleasure, and deviation were agents of death.

These distortions in the analysis of what came to be an epidemic greatly influenced government decisions about public health policies. Initially, the official position, repeated by a series of health ministers, classified the HIV epidemic as a kind of second-class epidemic. Or it was asserted that because it affected only minority groups of the population—sectors that were defined either as marginal or, paradoxically, as elite—the epidemic was of no fundamental importance. The worst aspect of this approach was the counterargument that because the country was suffering from traditional epidemics that could not be dealt with, it would almost be a luxury to tackle a minor epidemic that was of no social importance.

Even today, it is not uncommon to hear absurd discussions about which disease—HIV, tuberculosis, leprosy, malaria, and so on—should be selected as a priority. In reality, bureaucracy has already made its decision: the division responsible for the HIV and AIDS programme in the Ministry of Health ranks very low within the government's organizational structure. It has little political power. To give an idea of its relative insignificance, the country's president who took power in March 1990 never mentioned HIV or AIDS, and the director of the STI/AIDS division was unable to obtain an audience with him.

The cumulative effect of all these omissions, lack of interest, neglect, and incompetence was the creation of a body of incomplete or distorted information about HIV. This misleading information prevails both among the public, leading to panic and disturbances, and, lamentably, among health professionals themselves. It is not unusual for hospitals to refuse to accept seropositive patients, arguing that they will be unable to prevent infection of other patients or of health workers.

The failure of the public hospital network in Brazil, the catastrophic condition of health care, the ridiculously high cost of private health treatment in a country where 68 per cent of the population is living in poverty, and the profound disregard for the basic human rights of persons living with HIV are beginning to constitute a disaster of uncontrollable proportions. For many years, many have predicted that this scenario would occur if relevant HIV prevention and treatment policies were not introduced. Nothing was done, and the situation is getting worse.

In addition to the vast amount of suffering and the sharp increase in premature deaths, this lack of care places society as a whole in a state of some perplexity. And perplexity is a very poor counsellor. Rather than drawing up effective policies, officials respond—in a spirit of pity or in a welfare approach—by attempting to mitigate the most severe cases while failing to address the foreseeable deterioration of the situation as a whole. This picture illustrates the absence of a global strategy for confronting the HIV epidemic. Without projects, without programmes, without integration of the government and the community, without dissemination of information on prevention, without incentives for research, without epidemiological follow-up, all the actions taken are proving misdirected, incomplete, fragile, and conducive to prejudice and discrimination.

The indecisiveness of the Brazilian government's actions will certainly have devastating consequences. The country will reap the fruits of this incompetence in the form of a tragedy whose cost will be unbearable, either in economic or in human terms. There is no index that can be used to measure the suffering and grief that will result from these omissions.

To sum up the Brazilian picture, I would like to emphasize that alongside the tragedy of abandonment and lack of care is the question of human rights. This is at the centre of a world-wide challenge to HIV. The more disorganized and ineffective the programmes to combat this epidemic, the more widespread social discrimination becomes, condemning people living with HIV to social death. I have observed that the tendency toward secrecy, the paranoid flight from their own disease, is destroying the quality of life for people living with HIV. They are subjected to shame, fear, and guilt, which prevent them from objectively choosing forms of therapy that are appropriate to their cases. Many opt for a crude form of social nonexistence. They give up on the idea that they are citizens with acquired rights. Moreover, they become secretive even with their sexual partners.

This secrecy, in its obsessive forms—and I am not referring to privacy here—has been one of the things that enable the virus' spread. The self-awareness of persons living with HIV is an essential tool for bringing about the changes in behaviour that are capable of halting the advance of the virus. But public policies that encourage fear, shame, guilt, and secrecy are the epidemic's accomplices.

This is the form of war that is being waged on Brazilians—a war that is not directed against the epidemic but that attacks seropositive persons instead. This war, full of mystifications, has dominated the Western world in recent years. The result is that many of us who are living with the disease recognize ourselves as being the battlefield in an unsuccessful war against a death that Western civilization has decided to classify as obscene.

In the face of the world's war against AIDS, we have to become recalcitrant—for reasons of civil disobedience and passive resistance; for the sake of political action that runs counter to the policy of piously condemning us to social death. As a political act, I want to be impertinent by not clinging to ultimate truths and by doubting, searching, and singing hymns to life. I am a conscientious objector in a cowardly war that needs to be wiped from the face of the earth.

The Look of the Times

One experience I imagine I share with others living with HIV is that at any public meeting, when I say that I have AIDS, all those present inevitably look at me in the same way. They give me a look that says that I am the one who is marked for death. We are all going to die, the collective attitude seems to say, but you, the one with AIDS, are most marked for death.

This look is not characteristic of a specific group or of a specific occasion. It is the look of the age. Undeniably, the 1980s have chosen the seropositive—whether or not they have the disease—as our age's prime example of those who are optimally marked for death.

I do not think that this look is the look of prejudice. The type of prejudice that implies that a person living with HIV has decided to die views things differently. It is a prejudice that treats the concept of being marked for death as an ethical option that values death as something definitive—something that supplants social death and establishes the present as indicative of the act of dying. The look of prejudice is the voyeurism of discrimination that summarily defines AIDS solely as a contagious, incurable, and fatal disease, without explaining that infection by HIV can be avoided, since we know how it is transmitted. And although the virus cannot be removed from the body, the infection may be treatable.

The "look of the age" is the collective recognition of the broken promises of the twentieth century: the promise of eternal life offered by medical technology, the promise of the good life and everlasting youth offered by advertising, the promise of guilt-free sex without consequences given by the illusions of sexual freedom. This look of the age, which singles me out as marked for death, is a symptom of an uneasy conscience, an embryonic manifestation of what should be the awareness of HIV as the crisis of our civilization.

It is difficult to meet this look of the age and to counter it with the look of what I call life in the face of death. Faced with this look, one has to avoid the temptation of attributing truth to the words of the dying man on his deathbed, who has the right to say whatever he wants because of his complicity in the mystery of the beyond. In fact, I know nothing about life after death. If AIDS inspires me to ask any question, it is the following: what life, if any, exists before death?

Any possible complicity we want, in order to speak our piece about seropositives, must derive from the permanent mystery of life. This truth, which is brought out by the disease, reminds us that a person living with AIDS is not a half citizen, or the wreckage of a citizen, but rather a citizen in a special situation. Precisely because this person is not shipwrecked on the shores of productive society, he or she is also not above good and evil. His or her enemies, where both discrimination and exile are concerned, are piety and self-pity, pity and a refusal to become involved. Strength can come only from critical and self-critical awareness.

If a person living with AIDS passively accepts being a visual percept of the look of the age, any relationship he or she establishes is a trap. When he or she enters into a therapeutic relationship with someone purely as a visual percept, it is done without meeting the other's gaze with his or her own as agent. This two-way visual exchange is of equal value when relating to doctors, therapists, friends, and traditional medical practitioners—in short, to all those around us.

I can say without fear of being too far wrong that there is a certain comfort in accepting the gentle gaze directed on us by those who love us and have chosen us as marked for death. We are flattered by a ceremony at which the deceased is present, and it is much more disturbing for the officiants than for the living corpse. However, the price to be paid for this comfort is that of conformism. It is a road of no return to the harshest regions of social death. For my part, I decided that I preferred to be an inconvenient corpse. A well-behaved corpse lets itself be buried right away, with a few candles and tears.

Time of War

Disease has been explained in ways that associate all pathological processes with internal wars between the body and an external enemy. Certainly, the vitality of these metaphors stems from the fact that microbiology was born at a time in Western history when nationalism was gaining strength, when its brutal and lasting wars were breaking out. Western medicine became, despite its humanitarian message, a powerful instrument of war. The predominance of the image of disease as war varies from disease to disease. With HIV, the war has reached a mystical point. In the developed countries, HIV emerged at a time when infectious diseases were no longer considered serious medical problems, and one of the victories of advanced medical technology was increased life expectancy.

HIV came as an irrational challenge. It led to a major upheaval in the theory of Western medicine. It associated sex with death. And not just any sex, but the deviant sex of gays, a group whose coming out had revolutionized the scientific concepts of sexuality. And not just any death, but a death that involved a total breakdown of the body, without any explosion or any act of heroism or acute violence—an ugly, deforming, medieval death.

It does not matter that the epidemic quickly demonstrated that its history was unrelated to the prejudiced patterns of the much-publicized, obscurantist ideology of risk groups. The disease remained, in the world's imagery, an enigma. A common language in the world press, even among major scientists, made AIDS an insoluble mystery. Many people spoke of the disease with a certain humility, saying that it drastically undermined the traditional arrogance of medicine. In addition to the scientific revelation of a mysterious, infectious, incurable, and fatal disease, a new mythology was being born. A war was being waged against an all-powerful enemy possessing almost magical powers.

These metaphors of a mysterious war are modern, or postmodern, versions of the myth of the Fall and Salvation. HIV as a mystery presupposes blame, a victim, or perdition. And its solution calls for a hero, a saviour, or a supreme power. In this way, the incurability and the mortality of HIV came to incorporate metaphysical elements in its pathology. The mystery lay in the patient. The cure, the element of salvation, was part of the miracle. Medicine was assigned the prominent role of saviour. Once installed as a mystery, HIV becomes a lost battle for people whose assigned role is that of the vehicle of original sin. As victims to be saved, they are thus prepared to submit to every type of therapeutic dictatorship.

Is there any possible solution? Perhaps there is, by simply saying that HIV is a disease like any other. This approach involves a policy of prevention, which, in my view, is the issue that will dominate the 1990s. Such a policy must be based on the affirmation that we all must learn to live with HIV.

Within this picture of ambiguously defined mystical distortions, in which HIV became a war between good and evil, the basic formula for the ideological framework was the synthesis AIDS = DEATH. One of the first symbols used in information programmes on HIV was disseminated by the World Health Organization. It showed two hearts, romantically intertwined, with the intersection of these organs of affection forming the almost medieval image of a skull. It was succeeded, worldwide, by vigorous publicity campaigns in which, alongside health warnings, there was a proliferation of images of tombs, crosses, coffins, withered flowers, and dead bodies.

We continue to be subjected to imagery based on the supertechnological wars that took place at the end of this century—missiled, push-button wars in which soldiers who rarely faced one another were mutilated inside the armour of highly sophisticated equipment. With HIV, the patient becomes the battlefield, the landscape that dehumanizes his or her own emotional structure and will to live.

When I fell ill, I realized that I was not a battlefield. This was not a war, with victors and vanquished, but a lack of harmony between beings with different objectives. I developed an ecological metaphor for myself. And I saw preservation as the result of harmony and not of war, balance as the result of work and not of violence, preservation as the result of inventiveness and veneration for the real world. I created for myself a need for peace, a state diametrically opposed to passivity. There was a time when I criticized my need for solitude, born of the fear of death. I made my strong fear of death into a bridge to the pleasure of living with others. I came to understand that I am legion. I am one of many. I felt as if the entire world were flowing through my bloodstream. And I wanted to understand this more, in order to better share this one earth with those many human beings whom we bring to life.

The Present Time

In my inner vocabulary, I say that I constantly confront the virus without any imagined fear, but also without any optimistic illusions. We are staring at each other, the virus and I. Whoever blinks first loses. It may blink first, seductively and with an air of complicity. I am going to keep my eyes open. What I see is that to live today is, among other things, to live with HIV. I see this as part of my responsibility to myself, to my survival, and to those living with me.

If there is a cure for this epidemic, it will involve a recovery and reintegration of power. Our civilization separated us from our bodies, making them mere productive machinery. It separated us from pleasure, turning it into a consumer commodity. It separated us from awareness, turning it into feelings of guilt, shame, and fear. It separated us from experience and time, turning these into a succession of empty moments. It separated us from space, turning it into a mutilated environment. The HIV epidemic is a tragic part of the evolution of these separations.

I have learned that I am many, that I too am humankind, such as it is. I have come to understand that what makes us a human whole is not the aspects in which we are identical but precisely the differences that make for conflicts, disagreements, and distances among human beings. This is what unites us, through a primitive and insuperable force: solidarity. And my definition of solidarity is precisely that ability to recognize and rejoice in difference, to see ourselves in the eyes of others and recognize that they are different from us and yet as human as we are.

I believe that we all have a right to our privacy, to secrecy, anonymity, and so on. But we do not have any right to abandon others. That could be described as a crime, as a deliberate failure to help those who are in danger. Much of the uneasy silence among people who think that talking about HIV means discussing pathology and cure stems from violent prejudices that will have disastrous consequences. We need to describe, to denounce, to claim, to give free rein to hope.

I know that a great deal of clarification is going to be needed so that the story of this epidemic can one day be told as an example of the failure of our civilization. The politics, the ignorance, the hypocrisy, the prejudices, the vanity, the lies, the complicity with evil, the silence, the moral anaesthesia, the insensitivity—I am becoming increasingly certain that the sum of society's responses to HIV will have far more serious consequences than the virus' own capacity for extermination. I am not yet sure what we will inherit from HIV. But we need to be alert to the kind of heritage we will pass on to the postcure era. Yes, a cure for the virus will arrive. Until then, we need to listen attentively to the confused testimony of our times.

The experience of HIV is not purely the experience of physical pain or of physical extermination, as it is often pictured. The first experience of this epidemic is one of immense moral pain that goes to the very heart of the political and poetic struggle of our century's tragedy. The only global cure for this pain is solidarity, a broad movement capable of denying the melodrama and capturing the movement of the epidemic's tragedy. Long live life!

Appendix: UNDP HIV-Related Language Policy

Language and the images it evokes shape and influence behaviour and attitudes. The words used locate the speaker with respect to others, distancing or including them, setting up relations of authority or of partnership. Language affects listeners in particular ways, empowering or disempowering, estranging or persuading, and so on. The use of language is an ethical and a programmatic issue.

UNDP has adopted the following principles to guide its HIV-related language.

Language should be inclusive and not create or reinforce a Them/Us mentality or approach.

> For example, a term like "intervention" places the speaker outside of the group of people for or with whom he or she is working. Words like "control" set up a particular type of distancing relationship between the speaker and the listeners. Care should be taken with the use of the pronouns "they," "you," "them," and so forth.

It is better if the language used is drawn from the vocabulary of peace and human development rather than from the vocabulary of war.

> For example, synonyms could be found for words like "campaign," "control," and "surveillance."

Descriptive terms used should be those preferred or chosen by the persons described.

For example, "sex workers" is often the term preferred by those concerned rather than "prostitutes"; "people living with HIV" and "people living with AIDS" are preferred by infected persons rather than "victims" or "patients."

Language should be value neutral, gender sensitive, and empowering rather than disempowering.

Terms such as "promiscuous," "drug abuse," and all derogatory terms alienate rather than create the trust and respect required. Terms such as "victim" or "sufferer" suggest powerlessness; "haemophiliac" or "AIDS patient" identifies a human being by his or her medical condition alone. "Injecting drug users" is used rather than "drug addicts." Terms such as "living with HIV" recognize that an infected person may continue to live well and productively for many years.

Terms used need to be strictly accurate.

For example, "AIDS" should be used only to describe the conditions and illnesses associated with the significant progression of infection. Otherwise, the terms used include "HIV infection," "HIV epidemic," "HIV-related illnesses or conditions," and so on. "Situation of risk" is used rather than "risk behaviour" or "risk group," since the same act may be safe in one situation and unsafe in another. The safety of the situation has to be assessed each time.

The terms used need to be adequate in order to inform accurately.

For example, the modes of HIV transmission and the options for protective behaviour change need to be explicitly stated so as to be clearly understood within all cultural contexts.

The appropriate use of language respects the dignity and rights of all concerned, avoids contributing to the stigmatization and rejection of the affected, and assists in creating the social changes required to overcome the epidemic.

Index